**Mark G Bowditch**

**Damian R Griffin**

# ON-THE-JOB

# TRAINING

# FOR

# SURGEONS

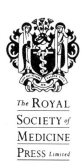

The ROYAL
SOCIETY of
MEDICINE
PRESS Limited

A   P R A C T I C A L   G U I D E

I Wimpole Street, London WIM 8AE, UK
16 East 69th Street, New York, NY 10021, USA

**British Library Cataloguing in Publication Data**
A catalogue record for this book is available from the British Library
ISBN 1-85315-314-1

Cartoons by Graham Hagan, Charing, Kent
Design by Elizabeth Fuller, Leighton Buzzard, Bedfordshire
Phototypeset by Dobbie Typesetting Limited, Tavistock, Devon
Printed in Great Britain by Ebenezer Baylis, The Trinity Press, Worcester

# CONTENTS

# FOREWORD

The 1990s have seen a number of radical changes in surgical education including a reduction in the length of training and a new emphasis on explicit teaching rather than learning by observation. At the same time pressure on service delivery may lead people to feel that there is no time for carefully prepared and planned education. Thus there is a need to integrate training as closely as possible with service delivery so that the patient's interests are not sacrificed to the needs of surgical education.

Alongside the changes in surgical education, there has been a rapid growth in educational research in the area of professional education. It is excellent to see a book which takes account of both these factors and one which has been written by a team combining expertise in professional and teacher education in Professor Hargreaves with the recent experience of Mark Bowditch and Damian Griffin as surgical trainees. At The Royal College of Surgeons of England we have recognised the importance of training those delivering surgical education by developing our own 'Training the Trainers' courses and this has made us aware of how many people involved in surgical training would welcome practical advice and guidance on on-the-job training. This book therefore fills an important gap.

The book contains much for everyone involved in surgical training. It is aimed at trainees and trainers but I think it will also appeal to people with a more general interest in medical education. Surgical tutors, for example, will find plenty of ideas to apply to their educational role while medical educators and trainers in specialties other than surgery will recognize the commonalities underlying all training of this type. The book focuses on the relationship between the trainer and the trainee and on the process required for successful on-the-job training. In this way it complements other recent publications, including distance learning courses, with their emphasis on the acquisition of the knowledge which underpins surgical skills. If you are a trainee you will find it contains useful information on topics such as negotiating training plans, questioning techniques, receiving feedback and reflecting critically on what you have learnt. If you are a trainer, these topics can provide a stimulus to reviewing the model you use for training. The authors' aim is to move away from the model of training by 'osmosis' towards one of partnership. Many of us will recognize the weaknesses of the old model from our own experience as surgical trainees and I welcome the book's emphasis on the rights and responsibilities of both trainer and trainee within the partnership.

**Professor JD Hardcastle**
Senior Vice President, Royal College of Surgeons of England

v

# PREFACE

This Guide begins with the challenge of a new approach to surgical training. The surgical Royal Colleges have taken up the challenge and introduced innovative distance learning and surgical skills programmes; postgraduate deans have joined their surgical colleagues and the Colleges in providing local infrastructures for the new training. But the essential part of learning to be a surgeon continues to be the experience and training that takes place at the coalface; at the workplace; at the cutting edge; at the battle front — there are many metaphors, but all mean 'on the job'.

The Guide comes from a major research project undertaken in hospitals in Anglia and demonstrates the value of asking education experts from another discipline, whose members can look at learning without the burden of baggage that comes from the medical teaching tradition. We have learned a great deal in Cambridge in the process of this research and I am delighted that practical results are being made available to surgical trainees and their trainers wherever the challenge of the new training is taken up.

**John SG Biggs**
Postgraduate Dean
January 1997

# INTRODUCTION

## The challenge

Following the Calman reforms and the New Deal, the training time from appointment as a Senior House Officer (SHO), through the Specialist Registrar grade, to the taking up of a consultancy is to be much reduced — a shorter working week over fewer years. So the quality and quantity of training needs to be improved. This Guide is designed to meet the changing needs and demands for training that now impinge on SHOs, Specialist Registrars and Consultants in surgical specialties.

What is to be done?

> We need to look again at how doctors learn and how teaching methods can be improved in order that time spent in education can be used efficiently. Supervision and feedback are crucial . . . The integration of theoretical teaching with practical work, progressive assessment and feedback to teachers and trainees are essential.
>
> Sir Kenneth Calman, Chief Medical Officer, 1993[1]

## Is there a problem?

Concern about the quality of training has a long history.

> In only one respect has there been a decided lack of progress in the domain of medicine, that is in the time it takes to become a qualified practitioner. In the good old days a man was turned out thoroughly equipped after putting in two winter sessions at a college and spending his summers in running logs for a sawmill. Nowadays it takes anywhere from five to eight years to become a doctor. It seems odd that a man should study eight years now to learn what he used to acquire in eight months.
>
> Stephen Leacock, economist and humorist, 1910
>
> No progress has as yet been made towards formulating the concept of the clinician as teacher. It is still supposed that because a man is an accomplished physician he is an excellent teacher. Clinical teaching in London remains an incident in the life of a busy consultant.
>
> Abraham Flexner, reformer of medical education, 1910

It is widely recognised that the outcomes of British postgraduate medical training are good. The degree of junior doctors' satisfaction with the process of training in more recent times is, however, variable. Several surveys indicate that many juniors are critical of some of the ways in which they are trained.

EVALUATIONS OF POSTGRADUATE TRAINING

Formally defined teaching rounds for PGME are uncommon . . . Most consultant PGME teaching appears to be provided in general ward rounds (business rounds). The teaching element is rarely defined . . . There is relatively little formal teaching in outpatients . . . For the majority of trainees, educational opportunities within outpatients were *ad hoc* . . . The most common criticism levelled by trainees was that they did not have the opportunity to examine, treat and learn about complex cases . . . Overall, there is little scheduled teaching in theatres. On the whole, trainees learn by assisting the consultant but this relies heavily on the willingness of the individual surgeon to teach . . . [2]

Most trainees want more and better training. Under 10% believe training is given a high priority by their seniors. Some believe more use could be made of registrars in the training of SHOs and that their existing contribution could be better recognised. Many trainees receive little feedback on progress in training. The feedback provided tends to be sparse, haphazard, implicit and indirect.[3]

The responses obtained to the questionnaire indicate the large extent to which SHOs are in a grade which includes training only in name. The finding is largely consistent across all survey specialties and hospital types . . . This paper shows that there is very little systematic teaching, few available good teachers and that learning is very much an ad hoc process . . . Just over half the SHOs cited registrars or senior registrars as providing some teaching... That only about half of SHOs cite consultants as providing most of their teaching is dramatic and a figure for concern . . . SHOs opted for senior registrars and registrars as their preferred teachers rather than consultants.[4]

## Towards a solution of the problem

Following the Calman reforms, the introduction of the BST for 2 to 3 years, leading to the MRCS (or AFRCS), should lead to a broader and better basic education for surgeons in this grade. For specialist registrars, the higher surgical training (HST) lasting between 4 and 6 years and leading to the CCST, should also enhance the quality of training. Improvement in the quality of formal training at all levels, welcome as this will be, does however raise the issue of how well the formal and on-the-job training are articulated with each other, so that they are mutually supportive. Better formal training will raise expectations both of better on-the-job training and of better ways of linking the two so that training as a whole becomes more coherent and so more effective.

x

## THE NEW TRAINING

A feature of the new training is the emphasis on rigorous assessment of progress against defined criteria . . . Evidence that effective training has taken place will lead to recognition of the trainee's competence and skill and a recommendation to the appropriate authority that a certificate of completion of specialist training should be awarded. . . . An aspect that will be new to many is the introduction of training agreements between the trainee, postgraduate dean, and the hospital trust(s) where training is to take place . . . Key elements [include] the structure and aims of the teaching programme and the standards of achievement expected of the trainee; an explanation of the methods and frequency of assessment; a commitment by consultants to regular in-service tuition; and protected time for trainees to study and be trained. There will also be a commitment from the trainee to take an active part in the training.[5]

Because the training period will be shorter, and educational standards must be maintained, the training element in all training grade posts must be strengthened. Service work done must complement training rather than interfere with it. . . . Education and training at SHO level is experimental learning while working in a health care team and providing a clinical service. However, it must be the right kind of service, with appropriate supervision, an opportunity to reflect on learning and a structured system to identify and support progress . . . Most learning takes place opportunistically in the context of practising medicine. The SHO needs to work within their own level of competence, and appropriate supervision should be readily available to advise, assist and educate.[6]

Junior doctors see on-the-job training — where training is combined with, and runs alongside, service delivery — as important, and will doubtless continue to do so. Yet little has been written on how this is best done. The Guide explains how trainers and trainees can improve on-the-job training for surgeons.

The Guide:

- helps trainers (Consultants, Specialist Registrars) to train more effectively
- helps Consultants and Registrars to work as partners in training SHOs
- helps trainees (Specialist Registrars, SHOs) to get the best out of training.

Teaching can also help you to learn. When you teach, you test out and refine the quality and depth of your own knowledge, skill and understanding. The Guide helps Specialist Registrars to teach and to learn through teaching.

**xi**

The Guide is grounded in a research and development project, sponsored by the Postgraduate Dean and funded by the Anglia Postgraduate Medical and Dental Education Committee. The project sought to identify good practice in different specialties in different hospitals. Doctors who volunteered to take part in the project are among those committed to improving training, seeing the Calman reforms as a challenge and opportunity. We do not claim they are typical, but the settings and circumstances in which they work are to be found everywhere. Ideas developed during the project were tested out by volunteers. It is recognised that producing evidence beyond the testimony of those involved on the effectiveness of particular training practices is unusually exacting. Wherever possible Consultants, Registrars and SHOs speak in their own words to describe their experiences and their responses to training, both old and new. Naturally, they remain anonymous.

## References

1. Calman KC. Medical education: a look into the future. *Postgraduate Medical Education* 1993; **69** (supplement 2): S3–S5.
2. Barker A, Scotland AD, Challah S, Gainey B, Bayley IA. A comparative study of postgraduate medical education in North East Thames Region. *Postgrad Med J* 1994; **70**: 722–7.
3. Booth M, Bradley H, Hargreaves DH, Southworth GW. Unpublished survey of junior doctors, 1994.
4. Grant J, Marsden P, King RC. Senior house officers and their training. *BMJ* 1989; **299**: 1263–8.
5. Biggs J. New arrangements for specialist training in Britain: guidance notes for implementing the specialist registrar grade. *BMJ* 1995; **311**: 1242–3.
6. Committee of Postgraduate Medical Deans and UK Conference of Postgraduate Deans. *SHO training: tackling the issues, raising the standards*, 1995.

# HOW TO USE THE GUIDE

> *There is a profound gap between applicable and actionable knowledge. The former tells you what is relevant; the latter tells you how to implement it in the world of every-day practice.*
>
> Chris Argyris and Donald Schön, educationists, 1974

It is easy, on the basis of sound educational principles, to offer advice on how to improve the training of doctors in hospitals — e.g. trainers should give trainees more feedback. This is just applicable knowledge, which trainers may know and understand but with no noticeable impact on their training practices.

This Guide aims at actionable knowledge, which explains precisely how to implement the advice in the everyday life of a hospital — in theatres, clinics and wards.

The Guide is divided into four Parts.

**Part One and Part Four** deal with the **key ideas** — on-the-job training, osmosis and coaching, the meaning of progression, education and training.

**Part Two** describes the basic **techniques** of training — asking questions, explaining, giving feedback.

**Part Three** focuses on the **settings** where you put these training techniques into action — operating theatres, clinics and wards.

Select sections according to your interest rather than reading from cover to cover.

## How TRAINERS might use the Guide

The ideal way to use this Guide is when all the Consultants in a department:

- commit themselves to making training a high priority and to improving everybody's skills at both learning and teaching
- decide that they will use the Guide to help to change training practices
- involve the whole department, Consultants, Specialist Registrars and SHOs and all other professional staff with the aim of creating a training culture

- treat Specialist Registrars both as trainees and, under the supervision of the Consultants, as contributors to the training of the SHOs.

If the whole team shares the same goal, success will be achieved more quickly.

Skim read Parts One and Four, then focus on those Sections in Parts Two and Three which you believe will be most important to you. Section 10 discusses written training plans which may require agreement among all the trainers. Some parts of the Guide will simply reflect what you already do. Other parts will give you ideas for developing those aspects of training which you would like to improve.

Teaching in on-the-job training (OJT), like any other skill in medicine, takes time and practice to learn. You can no more read advice on how to train effectively and then immediately put it into successful practice than you can read about a surgical operation and then carry it out easily and with total success in theatre. Skill in teaching, as in operating, is best acquired step by step. So do what you did in learning to operate — focus on, and master, one aspect at a time.

Some Sections could be used, in whole or part, for a departmental discussion, in protected time for formal training, to discuss approaches to, and strategies for, OJT. Talking through the members' feelings and ideas about OJT is a good way of creating interest in improving its quality. All the Sections in Parts Two and Three can be used in this way, Sections 5 and 9 should provoke stimulating debate.

## How TRAINEES might use the Guide

As a junior doctor, you will use the Guide mainly to help you

- make the most of the on-the-job training offered to you
- learn how to identify more opportunities for learning within the daily routines of service delivery
- exploit those opportunities more fully by learning how to elicit better training from everyone you are working with.

You are advised to start by skim reading Sections 2 and 4 in Part One and then move to Section 5 on taking control of your learning. You will then probably pick out those Sections in Part Two (techniques) and Part Three (settings) that are of interest and relevance to you. You will find it useful to read Section 10, whether or not you have an official training plan, since some of the ideas there can help you plan your on-the-job learning for yourself.

Learning in OJT, like any other skill in medicine, takes time and practice to learn. You can no more read advice on getting the best out of training and then immediately put it into successful practice than you can read about a surgical operation and then go into theatre to carry it out easily and with total success. Skill in learning, as in operating, is best acquired step by step. So do what you do in operations — focus on, and master, one aspect at a time.

Choose **one** Section on which to work for a time. When you have made progress in that area, turn to another topic. It is impractical to work on all Sections at once.

## How 'TRAIN THE TRAINER' COURSE LEADERS might use the Guide

Such courses will increasingly be concerned with training trainers to be more effective in OJT as well as in formal training sessions. The Guide may be used:

● as a complement to work on various kinds of formal and off-the-job training
● as a resource for clarifying the nature of OJT and its theoretical and conceptual infra-structure (Parts One and Four)
● as a text or resource book for training sessions on OJT
● as the basis for designing activities and exercises on either the techniques of OJT or the application of the techniques in action settings.

## FOR ALL

Each Section ends with a set of Action Points, which may be treated as an *aide-memoire*, copied onto cards or into a filofax and be carried in a white coat pocket.

# I TRAINING AS APPRENTICESHIP — OSMOSIS OR COACHING?

*In postgraduate medical education, 'apprenticeship' is the accepted dominant model of training — defined as learning by doing under the supervision of an experienced practitioner . . . This model, if unanalysed, perpetuates the unhelpful confusion between training and service, to the extent that providing the service may become identified with receiving training . . . But learning by doing in the absence of a teacher to provide guidance and feedback, has the inherent potential of learning the wrong thing in the wrong way . . .*

J Grant, P Marsden and RC King, medical educators, 1989

*The term on-the-job training is one I abhor, because it generally implies that people will pick things up as they go along. We think, as we do in many cases of apprenticeships, that putting a young person with someone experienced will automatically transfer knowledge and theory. The developmental responsibility of the coach-manager is much broader than that.*

Sir John Harvey-Jones, industrialist, 1994

*How are skills learned? By experience. How, then, are they best taught? By coaching.*

Theodore Sizer, educationist, 1984

## THIS SECTION

● explains the difference between the two major models of apprenticeship
● describes the strengths of apprenticeship by coaching

In talking about training, doctors commonly use two words — 'osmosis' and 'apprenticeship'.

Osmosis refers to the vague processes by which, during the daily round of service delivery, a trainee somehow 'picks up' relevant knowledge, skills and understanding.

It is an unplanned and unsystematic yet pervasive feature of professional learning. Much is acquired simply by watching and listening to colleagues as well as directly through 'hands-on' experience. Osmosis includes modelling by the trainer and incidental learning where a trainee incidentally gains some knowledge or skill when primarily intending to reach some other goal. There is also coincidental learning when the trainee happens to be around as the Consultant encounters a rare condition.

I

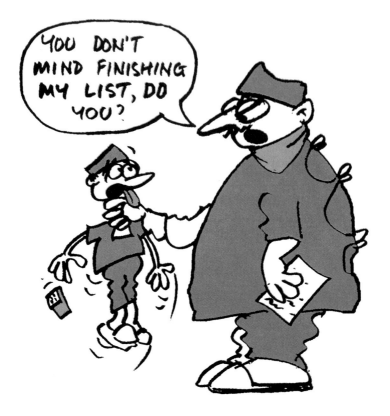

An apprenticeship model of training does not exclude elements of osmosis — learning simply by being around the trainer or imitating the trainer after a period of close observation. But true apprenticeship — a model of training widely adopted in a variety of professions and trades in the past — extends far beyond osmosis, for there is planned, systematic and deliberate teaching. 'Sitting next to Nellie' — the phrase often used to describe the industrial version of the osmotic apprentice-ship — becomes a more effective form of training when she takes her responsibilities seriously and willingly assumes an active role in shaping the apprentice's learning.

The effective 'master' traditionally coached the apprentice by:

- demonstrating knowledge and skill
- being a role model in how to relate to colleagues and clients
- providing lots of hands-on experience
- guiding the apprentice through regular practice
- setting clear objectives and targets to support the apprentice's learning

2

- supervising progression through the steps that lead to mastery
- having sufficient self-restraint to resist doing the job for the apprentice
- seeing the apprentice as a help to his/her own work, not as a hindrance to it
- accepting that a bright apprentice is a person the master can learn with and from.

If the surgeon trainer offers structured training that is intentional, planned in a sequence, monitored and followed up, it is the apprenticeship-by-coaching model. If it is not, then it is the unstructured and much inferior apprenticeship-by-osmosis, where the learning is unplanned, unsystematic and unsupported.

THE MERITS OF APPRENTICESHIP-BY-COACHING:
the views of some Consultant surgeons

*I learnt how to be a trainer by being trained the way I was trained. I learnt from people who stood there all the time training me — not only how to do the operation but how to train when it became my turn to train. Some people learn without much training. The trouble is they just learn to do the operation successfully, they don't learn how to teach it.*

*[My own training] was completely unsupervised. The philosophy of one of the consultants was that he wasn't interested in teaching, he hadn't been taught himself and that gradually I would pick it up.*

*I was well trained. It was important that the consultants actually took my training seriously. They took it as a major part of the commitment of their professional life. The environment was right. A certain element of structured progress, a preparedness to talk to the trainee and speak to him directly, having created an environment in which the trainee would accept that as not just an off-the-cuff comment, but as part of continued training and assessment. So that in criticising me one moment for something I'd done, I would know it wasn't a black mark against my career, but a part of trying to make me better. I might find an hour later a helpful comment was made. It was more guidance than criticism. That was the atmosphere created by all the consultants I worked for, that they were there to guide people — and their guidance extended to your domestic concerns and a general interest in what people did. Within that sort of atmosphere, criticism is taken in a positive way.*

*I was lucky in my surgical training at all stages. By chance I happened upon a senior registrar who was at the end of his days and didn't want to come in at night, wanted just to get his consultancy. He showed me the operations and left me to do them. I got lots of hands-on operating, which at the time was perfect for me. A friend, who was as talented, on the same training scheme got the reverse. He came into the job when the senior registrar was starting too. He learned nothing. The senior registrar hogged all the interesting cases. That's why I have a drive to improve juniors' training.*

## THE MERITS OF APPRENTICESHIP-BY-COACHING
### a psychological viewpoint

The coach seeks to provide active support to the trainee's learning. It is held by psychologists that there is an important space between what a learner is able to do independently and what he or she might do with the active support of, or in collaboration with, a more experienced person (the teacher). How the coach 'tells' or 'explains' or 'questions' matters in closing that space. Good teaching can serve as a kind of scaffolding around the skill or knowledge to be acquired, so that with its help, the trainee moves beyond what he or she could do alone. When the learning has been achieved through such help, the scaffolding can be removed: the teaching has been successful. Learning how to coach means learning how — through the teaching techniques adopted and the way they are put into practice — to provide scaffolding for the skills and knowledge that are, without help, just out of the apprentice's reach, but with help, within it.

Trainee surgeons, like all learners, experience the difficulty of applying what they know in an academic or intellectual sense. To transfer what they have learnt in books to clinical practice is not easily achieved through formal teaching sessions. On-the-job training, by contrast, is rich in possibilities for teaching by scaffolding for three reasons:

● it is in OJT that a trainer detects and documents that the trainee has only partially mastered a skill and needs help to develop it to the full

● it is in OJT that the trainer can then provide the scaffolding or active help by which the trainee is able to demonstrate the skill that could not have been done alone

● it is in OJT that the trainer can subsequently monitor the trainee's exercise of the skill and be satisfied that it is indeed mastered and that the scaffolding — and close supervision — is no longer required.

Getting trainee knowledge into effective practice through the coach's scaffolding is the most distinctive feature and greatest potential of OJT.

Some trainers perpetuate apprenticeship-by-osmosis on the grounds that if it was good enough for them it should be good enough for anybody. This argument ignores the fact that the knowledge, skills and techniques which trainees now have to acquire are greater than in the past and have to be acquired over a much shorter training period. Other trainers have evidently reacted critically towards their own training under the apprenticeship-by-osmosis model and have adopted a model in which the trainer is a coach. Some trainers have been trained under an apprenticeship-by-coaching model and want to continue with the approach to training they found so valuable.

4

# 2   UNDERSTANDING ON-THE-JOB TRAINING

> *When you're in a busy firm, your main agenda isn't to learn things, it's to get the work done.*
>
> Trainee, 1996
>
> *Until proper educational analysis of the contribution of service work to training is done, the enforced dominant model — of service being training — will persist.*
>
> J Grant, P Marsden & RC King, medical educators, 1989
>
> *All consultants have a part to play: the role of the majority will be to facilitate appren- ticeship learning through routine service work . . . Informal and opportunistic learn- ing should be valued highly as an important component of the overall educational package available to doctors in training. . . It should be developed and supported to increase its educational effectiveness.*
>
> The Report of SCOPME, 1994
> (The Standing Committee on Postgraduate Medical Education)

## THIS SECTION
- **describes the different types of training**
- **explains why OJT needs to be:**
    - **— planned rather than opportunistic**
    - **— fusional rather than intrusive**
    - **— cyclical rather than fragmented**
    - **— an investment rather than a duty**

The types of training are:
- 'off-the-job' or formal training, and
- 'on-the-job' training (OJT), which is either informal or semi-formal

**Formal, off-the-job training** occurs when teaching and learning are the only activities being intentionally undertaken and neither is directly related to any current or ongoing service delivery or patient under treatment. Lectures, seminars and courses are obvious examples. Formal training usually occurs in a dedicated place e.g. a seminar room.

**OJT — informal training** — takes place with a real case during service, usually with the patient present. The main settings for OJT are theatres, wards and clinics.

**5**

OJT — semi-formal training — is triggered by real cases during service but diverges from the case at hand into broader issues. Semi-formal training occurs, for instance, on a teaching ward round when the trainer discusses with the firm issues of diagnosis or management which link to but are not directly related to the patient before them. In some semi-formal situations — a meeting prior to the ward round, a meeting to discuss trauma lists or to study patients' X-rays — the patients are not present.

Semi-formal situations are often seen by trainees as especially rich in opportunities for teaching and learning, mainly because the issues are seen as relevant to their practice and the lack of immediate pressure from the demands of service delivery provides the 'space' for discussion. A common example is when a trainee in clinic goes to get advice on how to manage a patient, and then through that short conversation gets some teaching as well as a solution to a service problem.

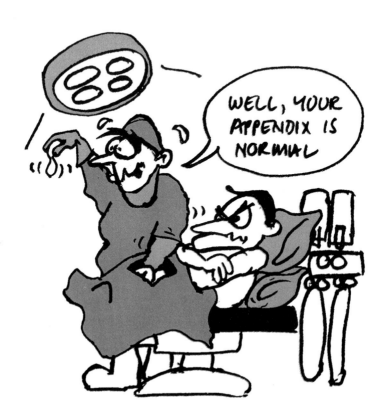

6

Apprenticeship-by-coaching involves a distinctive philosophy and set of practices. That is, OJT is:

- planned rather than just opportunistic
- fusional rather than intrusive
- cyclical rather than fragmented
- an investment rather than a duty.

These distinctions are explained below.

## Planned *versus* opportunistic OJT

Much of OJT has an opportunistic character. The trainer takes the line that training is contingent on the cases that turn up when the trainee is around to be taught and that there is sufficient time to engage in the teaching. Since, the argument runs, both variables are difficult to predict or control, trainee and trainer are destined to take a 'wait and see' line and make the most of any opportunities that arise.

From the perspective of apprenticeship-by-coaching, opportunistic OJT has several faults:

- it is a *re-active* rather than pro-active philosophy, inducing in both trainer and trainee a fatalism that they are at the mercy of events rather than the masters of them
- it underestimates the degree to which some aspects of both training and service delivery are predictable and open to control through planning
- it discourages both trainer and trainee from scanning service delivery for opportunities for OJT and then exploiting them in the interests of the trainee.

Planned OJT does not deny that OJT is indeed subject to service pressures and the chance of what turns up in the case load, but sees these as constraints upon training rather than as insurmountable barriers to it. OJT is not open to the kind of planning appropriate to formal training — deciding beforehand exactly what will be taught at what point in what sequence. OJT is, however, open to planning that is looser, more flexible and readily adaptable in the light of experience and changing circumstances.

How to design a training plan is the topic of Section 10, p. 69.

## Fusional *versus* intrusive OJT

Trainers and trainees often contrast training with service — one is doing either one or the other. This is natural enough for we put a mental frame round our actions in the light of our intentions. If we intend to teach, our action is framed as 'training': if we intend to treat patients, action is framed as 'service'.

### OJT in surgical training — a conceptual map

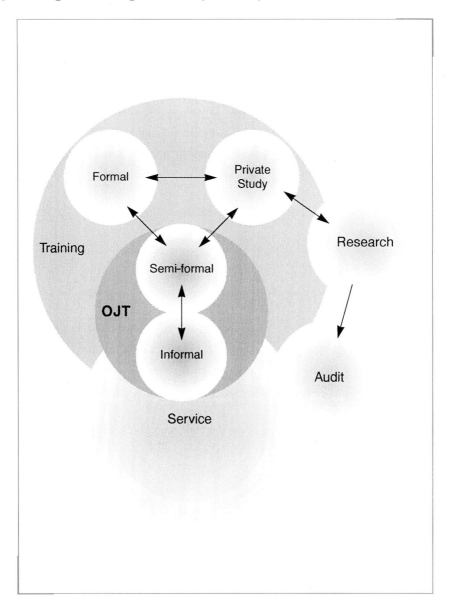

Sometimes training interrupts service delivery because the trainer, in order to teach, stops the service to start teaching (e.g. explains, or asks the trainee some questions, or demonstrates a skill to the trainee) and so takes longer to complete the service. As trainers rightly see such training as intrusive of service, they say there is insufficient time for training. On-the-job training is fine, the argument goes, but the job takes longer than it would otherwise do and that cannot be afforded.

OJT does not, however, always have to be intrusive. A second and far more significant form, which we might call fusional OJT, is when the OJT is fused with service, that is, the training is integrated, and takes place simultaneously, with service delivery. Intentions fuse, so frames fuse too. One is indeed doing two things at once.

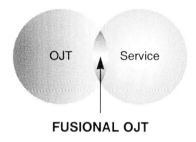

**FUSIONAL OJT**

In fusional OJT the job often takes no more time than if no training were taking place.

EXAMPLES OF FUSIONAL OJT

- a surgeon asks a trainee a question without stopping the surgery

- during a ward round a Consultant explains to the patient and the juniors present the nature of the treatment that has been selected

- the trainee who is seeking advice from the Consultant in clinic is asked to examine the patient in a way that allows the trainee to learn but does not require the trainer to make a separate or independent examination.

Fusional OJT is an efficient and effective form of OJT, but producing it in quantity and with quality is a highly skilled activity. There are two major components.

The first is the psychological change of abandoning the view that one can handle only one frame at a time — either teaching or service delivery. The two frames are

9

combined in fusional OJT. The coach moves from thinking or saying 'There just isn't enough time for teaching' to 'What opportunities are there in the next hour for any fusional OJT?' Every piece of service in which coach and trainee are co-present contains potential for fusional OJT.

The second component is the practical skill of learning how to insert the maximal amount of fusional OJT into service delivery and reduce intrusive OJT to a minimum.

Service is richer in opportunities for training than most trainers and trainees realise. Both coach and trainee have to learn how to scan the service in which they are jointly engaged, in order to recognise the opportunities and then exploit them to the full.

## Cyclical *versus* fragmented OJT

Ideally OJT has the structure of a coaching cycle with three phases.

PHASES OF A COACHING CYCLE

- a **planning phase** where coach and trainee decide the aspect of training on which to focus

- a **service phase** into which OJT is fused or blended

- a **follow-up phase** where coach and trainee review the quality of trainee performance and the training provided, and decide what to do in the next training cycle.

In practice, coaching cycles rarely take this ideal, cyclical form, since both the planning and follow-up phases are left out. The structure of OJT is often highly fragmented, and sometimes with good reason. Since some OJT is necessarily opportunistic, a formal planning phase is often not possible. In the same way, OJT often slides back into service delivery and there is neither the time nor the opportunity for any follow-up discussion — and sometimes no appropriate private place in which to conduct it.

## OJT as an investment versus training as a duty — training pays!

> *I'll be responsible in my lifetime for something like ten thousand operations. I could do ten thousand operations and die: what have I done? Not actually very much. If over twenty years I train ten guys over two years each, they too will do ten thousand opera- tions. And then if you could infuse them with the same ethic of teaching, it cascades like a chain letter.*
>
> Trainer
>
> *[The consultants] have our greater interest at heart and they seem to enjoy watching us mature, grow, improve, get better, get quicker. They get out of us keen, committed juniors. It's a trade-off. They get more skills, more work out of us and they in the long run save time by what they can do.*
>
> Trainee

The best planning is guided by a conception of training as an investment:

- a short-term investment — faster and better service delivery
- a long-term investment — a better Consultant in due course.

Training treated as a duty is a natural partner of OJT conceived as necessarily intrusive and opportunistic. But training can and should also be seen also as an investment, not merely in the self-evident sense of contributing to the development of the trainee, but also in the less obvious sense of making a highly effective contribution to current service delivery, including the work-load of the trainer.

In all aspects of surgery there are parts of operations — and cases in clinics and aspects of patient care on the ward — that are appropriately handed over to trainees. If the acquisition of some of the relevant knowledge and skill by trainees occurs very soon after their arrival in the firm or department, this frees the trainer to get on with those aspects of service that are too important or too difficult to be delegated.

Ensuring that trainees acquire some relevant knowledge and skills at a very early stage does require time and effort from the trainer, both to teach the relevant knowledge and skill and then to provide the close supervision to check that trainees can carry out the relevant clinical tasks effectively. But the trainer's time saved in subsequent weeks or months more than compensates for the initial outlay of trainer time. Moreover, trainees see that their training is being made a priority and that they are making speedy progress at an early stage. As a result their morale and confidence rise rapidly, which results in a more committed and competent trainee. Therefore, the investment in training pays off in several ways.

For training to be such a sound investment it has to be planned by the coach with great care. OJT occurs in a range of settings — theatres, wards and clinics — and a sound plan takes account of what can best be learned in one particular setting.

## Learning without coaching

The coach helps the trainee to learn, but this does not always mean that the coach must be engaged in teaching. It means, rather, that the coach ensures that the trainee is placed in conditions where learning can take place. The most obvious form of coaching in surgery is the teaching of operating skills in theatre, but there are other elements of training which have a different pattern. On-the-job learning by a trainee often occurs in conditions where the trainer is not even present.

Trainees must be in a position to profit from their own experience. Learning to recognise clinical conditions in patients and to make judgements about them, along continua such as normal-abnormal, common-rare, trivial-serious or super-ficial-extensive, requires exposure to many actual examples as well as text-book knowledge. Interpersonal skills, e.g. appropriate ways in which to relate to nursing and para-medical staff, or breaking bad news to patients or relatives, are learned through experience as well as observation of role models.

Coaches can help trainees to see the importance of learning through experience if they point out what can be learned in this way and in which settings. Work on wards and clinics can seem unduly boring to juniors if they ignore the fact that seeing common cases with high frequency (i) provides the essential background for recognising important variations of the condition and (ii) allows the mental processes underlying such recognition to move from being slow and analytical to becoming faster and more intuitive. Learning-on-the-job in the absence of explicit teaching is an important, but under-estimated, part of OJT.

# 3   THE PARTNERSHIPS IN COACHING

> The [trainee] cannot be taught what he needs to know but he can be coached.
>
> Donald Schön, educationist, 1987
>
> Trainees have to have confidence in their trainer. If they know it's like learning to ski or a trapeze act, if they know that if they fall I'm there, they'll jump.
>
> Consultant surgeon, 1996

## THIS SECTION
- **outlines the partnership between coach and trainee**
- **outlines the partnership between Consultant and Registrar as trainers**
- **outlines the responsibilities and rewards of being a coach and a trainee**

In apprenticeship-by-osmosis, the trainer leaves most of the responsibility for learning with the trainee. In apprenticeship-by-coaching, the trainer and trainee accept a range of responsibilities, but in turn receive significant rewards.

The **responsibilities of the coach** are:

- showing a real commitment to training
- taking the lead with trainees in making a plan for training and taking part in the plan's implementation
- supporting trainees through encouragement and by boosting self-confidence
- providing opportunities for learning that are appropriate to the trainee's needs
- taking a very active role in training by using a range of teaching methods
- giving feedback, both positive and negative
- helping the trainee to assess the rate and extent of progress in learning
- evaluating whether what was planned has in fact been achieved.

Unless these are evident, you cannot expect your trainees to be very committed either to the training or to the job itself. On-the-job training means that when the training is good the job also is done better.

The **rewards for the coach** are:

- a trainee who becomes effective faster
- a trainee who can be given greater day-to-day responsibility

- a trainee whose morale and self-confidence is high
- a trainee who respects the coach for first-class training.

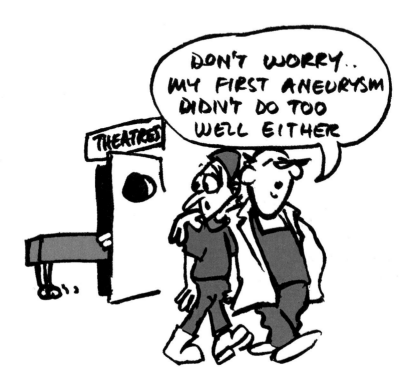

The **responsibilities of the trainee** are:

- a commitment to learning — being motivated
- a willingness to work hard through study and practice
- a responsive attitude to the coach's guidance and advice.

Unless these are evident, the trainee forfeits the right to expect much commitment from the trainer, and you cannot complain if the coach loses interest in you. It may not be enough for you to be committed: you have to show the trainer that you are — by taking an active interest in being taught. Your trainer will judge this, for example by whether you turn up for interesting operations or ask intelligent questions.

The **rewards for the trainee** are:

- receiving more teaching
- getting better at the job faster
- being trusted by the trainer and so being given more responsibility.

If a trainer is not very interested in your training, you may have to take diplomatic action to elicit more or better training — see Section 5, p. 21.

The partnership between Consultant and Specialist Registrar is essential to ensure the highest quality training for SHOs. Both play a coaching role, but the allocation of responsibilities should always be as explicit as possible, the roles should be complementary, and the contribution of the Specialist Registrar should remain under the supervision of the Consultant.

The **rewards of such a partnership** are:

- much more coherent training of the SHO
- the trainer becomes a more effective coach
- a 'training culture' that fosters learning is created
- the reputation for training leads to better applicants for junior posts.

---

- **Practise** as much as you can.
  A trainee surgeon needs constant cutting practice, a coach needs constant coaching practice.

- **Partnership matters**
  OJT is not something a trainer does to a trainee: it is a joint enterprise in which trainers and trainees co-operate to advance learning.

- **Progression** in coaching skills and progression in the knowledge and skills of surgery are both the outcome of practice combined with feedback from partners. In coaching as in surgery, you can't expect to improve without practice and feedback from partners.

---

# 4 PROGRESSION IN TRAINING

> *Coaching is an integral part of teaching the inexperienced of any age . . . A coaching relationship exists if someone seeks to move someone else along a series of steps, when those steps are not entirely institutionalised and invariant, and when the learner is not entirely clear about their sequence (although the coach is). The coach has to know when to force his man over a hurdle and when to let him sidle up to it . . . The coach may be rejected if he forces too fast a pace, especially at the outset. On the other hand, the pupil . . . may be lost to his mentor if the latter moves too slowly — lost through boredom, shattering of faith or other reasons.*
>
> Anselm Strauss, medical sociologist, 1969

## THIS SECTION

- **describes the steps of progression in surgical training**
- **explores how they apply in practice**

Coaching means moving the learner along a series of steps that are clear to the coach but as yet unclear to the trainee. For example, the steps of progression in the acquisition of operating skills may be charted as below.

## THE 7 STEPS OF PROGRESSION

- step 1: trainee observes (preferably with commentary from the coach)
- step 2: trainee assists the coach
- step 3: trainee does under the supervision of the coach (with full feedback)
- step 4: trainee does with the coach in the vicinity
- step 5: trainee does on his/her own
- step 6: trainee perfects it through regular practice and difficult /unusual cases
- step 7: trainee is now a teacher and teaches it.

These steps of progression can be adapted to apply to clinics and wards with only slight adaptation.

Progression means moving in an orderly, sequential way from step to step. The coach aids progression by arranging for learning opportunities that ease the

17

trainee's movement from one step to the next. In broad terms the steps at the heart of surgical training are a refinement of the 'see one, do one, teach one' maxim, a refinement which brings out the key role of the trainer.

For the trainee to gain the combination of confidence and competence that characterises the autonomous professional practitioner, the first five steps must be completed. Specialist Registrars towards the end of their 5 years, and new Consultants too, are at Step 6. Specialist Registrars may well be no further than Step 5 before assuming a teaching role with SHOs.

At any one time a trainee is not at the same step level for all aspects of training. For instance, a trainee may reach step 5 for the preparation and closing parts of an operation whilst being at step 2 for the central part.

> Early on I was taken through a few things with the bosses there from the beginning through to the end and then gradually they faded into the background and soon I was happily doing the first third and the last third of the operation. And then over the last fifteen months they've faded more and more from the scene in that I'm now doing some cases on my own, appropriate cases on my own, and I'm very happy with that.
>
> Trainee

The development of more explicit curricula and the specification of competences are clarifying what is involved in the staged transition from medical novice to Consultant.

New SHOs have on registration become competent however, they are once again novices with regard to the specialist training now to be acquired. At all stages in the movement from novice to consultant status, trainees will use the step approach, but for progressively more difficult tasks. Trainees quickly reach steps 5 or 6 for the simpler tasks, but remain at steps 1 or 2 for more complex skills.

A trainee is unlikely to pass through the steps at the appropriate rate if the trainer does not actively coach in a systematic way, monitoring carefully the step level of the trainee and then judging at what point and in which way the trainee must be moved to the next step. This includes accurate feedback from coach to trainees,

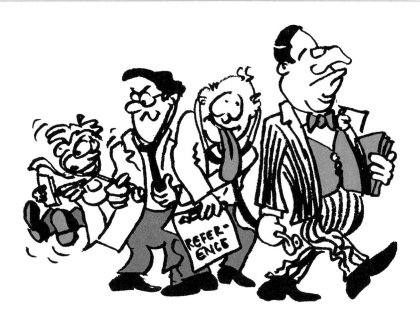

who otherwise may either believe they are not ready to move forward by under-estimating their own competence and achievement, or, by over-estimating their abilities, they seek to make progress before they are ready. Monitoring by the coach of trainee over- and under-confidence is a key to ensuring the proper progression by trainees.

Specification of the competences to be expected during each stage of training years is probably a precondition of ensuring more efficient and effective progression by trainees — see Section 10 on training plans.

Accurate self-assessment by trainees of their stage and step enhances progression, because it helps to focus trainee learning. The coach takes action either to check whether trainee self-assessment is accurate or to help the trainee develop the skill of accurate self-assessment. The assessments by both partners must be kept aligned.

# 5   TAKE CONTROL OF YOUR LEARNING — BE PRO-ACTIVE!

> *By teaching I mean the imparting of knowledge, and for that we are dependent on our teachers; by training I mean the cultivation of aptitude, and for that we are dependent on our opportunities and ourselves.*
>
> Wilfred Trotter, surgeon, 1932
>
> *It is as much the responsibility of the subordinate to manage his [coach] as of the [coach] to manage his subordinate.*
>
> Sir John Harvey-Jones, industrialist, 1994
>
> *Trainees will learn best when they see educational opportunities in every clinical situation.*
>
> The Report of SCOPME, 1994
> (The Standing Committee on Postgraduate Medical Education)

## THIS SECTION:
- **explains to trainees how being pro-active helps to elicit teaching from your trainer**
- **shows that being pro-active and taking the initiative with your learning is a skill you can learn and not an immutable personality characteristic**
- **illustrates how to be pro-active and take the initiative in effective ways**

Consultants with juniors partly or wholly funded by Postgraduate Deans have an obligation to provide training. Trainees are obliged to be committed to learning and to play an appropriate role as trainee.

In practice, formal obligations and good intentions with regard to training often fall foul of the daily grind. The demands of service on both trainers and trainees frequently distract both parties from the rich possibilities of OJT. Indeed, service is always in danger of squeezing out OJT. If trainees view their training passively and assume that the initiative always lies with trainers, then many opportunities for training remain unexploited. To be pro-active is:

- taking an active role in shaping training, not passively accepting what turns up
- taking the initiative to elicit teaching from trainers, not passively waiting for it
- being ready to ask questions of the trainer, not just answer them
- suggesting possible solutions to problems, not saying 'I don't know what to do'

**21**

- keeping your eye open for situations from which you might learn something e.g. an interesting or unusual case or operation
- asking to be present at and/or participate in work which is not part of your duty
- bouncing back when being pro-active and taking the initiative has not worked out for you.

Some trainees do these things more naturally or readily than others. One consultant divided trainees into three kinds:

- those who are diffident, take too little initiative and are uncomfortable about being pro-active — the '**wall-flower**'
- those who never miss a chance to learn, but are pro-active in a way that does not alienate the trainer — the '**fly-trap**'
- those who are so pushy they become a nuisance — the '**bramble**'.

This Section is particularly addressed to trainees who fall at the diffident end of the spectrum — feeling that being pro-active runs against the grain of their personality.

Consider first what juniors in the middle of the spectrum from 'wall-flower' to 'bramble' say.

PRO-ACTIVE TRAINEES — 'FLY-TRAPS'

*If you want to learn something, you have to get someone to teach you and you have to ask.*

*You learn very quickly to go and get training in the sense that you badger Consultants to tell you why they do things. You've got a particular problem and you badger them to give you some advice. They're very willing to give it. And it turns you into a more pro-active person: you don't want to be spoon-fed.*

*You have to be seen to be wanting to do things, to be asking to do things. You don't 'show' by being very quiet and staying in the corner and expecting things to be handed to you. You have to push to some extent.*

*Juniors say, 'I want to learn how to do this' and they go out and they push and they seek. The Consultant finds juniors coming up and saying, 'You're doing this on your list — can I do it, please?' He says, 'Oh yes, fine.' The Consultant can show them how to do it.*

Trainees at the diffident end of the spectrum approach their training differently.

## NON-PROACTIVE OR 'DIFFIDENT' TRAINEES

*I tend not to be a forceful and pushy person. I feel embarrassed to ask the Consultant questions. I don't want to upset him or make myself look stupid.*

*I don't think I could ask to do some operating. I'm not that sort of a person. I'm a bit retiring in some ways. If you ask me to do something, I'll always do it, but it's different asking you. I'm not built that way.*

Such trainees will get more out of their training if they think of being pro-active not as a fixed personality characteristic they lack but as a skill or technique for getting **what is rightfully theirs** — some solid OJT. Being pro-active is an aspect of the trainee's partnership with the coach. Some trainers will 'give away' some operating to ensure that trainees acquire experience, but most do not to the extent that trainees would like — sometimes with good reason, of course. As one trainee explains:

*Few trainers will say 'We're doing [a given] operation today. What would you like to do?' Any decent trainee has to say 'Do you mind if I do the operation today with you assisting me?' A trainee has to push himself forward to get the experience.*

Being pro-active is not just about getting hands-on experience but shaping the teaching that goes with it. As a coach explains to a trainee:

*If you're more pro-active, you'll get more teaching. It also means that if you're pro-active and that gets you more teaching, the teaching is going to be directed at the things you ask about or that you push towards. Since you know what you know and what you don't know, you know what you wish to know better than any of us, so you can direct us down the track you want to go. If you're just a passive learner, if you sit back and wait for it to come to you, much of what you're taught may be irrelevant, or a duplication of things you already know, or over your head. Whereas if you're pro-active, you're driving the learning, and it's more likely to be what you need to know. Concentrate on being pro-active. It's a very important aspect of your learning. We're going to be teaching you, but you're the person who's learning and there should be at least an equal balance of control over that process.*

At the other extreme of the pro-activity spectrum, trainees are pro-active to the point of being a nuisance to the trainer — 'brambles':

- are constantly badgering trainers with questions and requests
- ask thoughtless questions, the first that come into their heads, and ask them at the wrong moment
- ask for operating experience before they are ready, because they think that having merely seen one entitles them to do it entirely on their own
- 'try to run before they can walk' — through a mixture of poor self-assessment, over-confidence in themselves and under-assessment of the difficulties in surgery.

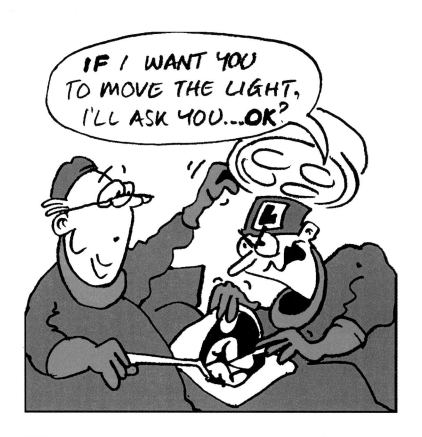

*This guy was a pain to teach. He would choose inappropriate times for coming to you with problems. He would come to me with a problem, see me dashing in and out of my office, and say, 'Can I have a minute of your time' and I'd yell 'What!?' He'd ask for some hands-on experience when it was completely inappropriate and if he'd thought about it he'd have realised it for himself. And then there was another trainee who kept asking me questions but he didn't really want to know the answer, just show-off questions. You'd give him something to do and he didn't do as he was asked. He thought doing the scuff work was beneath him. Some trainees want to acquire rather than learn — they want to acquire the fact that they've been to this hospital, that they got an FRCS, that they've done this, that and the other operation. And then there are very different trainees, those who are in the right place at the right time with the most appropriate question and answer, they're appreciative of being taught and you can tell they are learning.*

## Putting pro-activity into action

It requires some experience and some confidence to be pro-active in the best way, but it can be done if trainees:

- scan all service for opportunities for training and be ready pro-actively to seize the initiative
- ask to be taught by the coach at appropriate times
- learn to be pro-active by doing it in small ways where the trainer is almost certain to agree
- are pro-active in matters where they can prove they are ready to be given the responsibility
- choose situations with good chances that a request will be granted e.g. where there is not too much time pressure on the trainer
- recognise that learning to do an operation is a slow process best achieved by doing the easy parts under supervision and progressing to the more difficult parts before being ready to do the whole operation
- adopt a 'win some, lose some' philosophy and convince themselves they will not feel snubbed or upset if their request is refused.

Trainers help trainees make more of their learning opportunities in OJT when they actively encourage them to be pro-active and teach them the skill, including how to avoid being diffident or excessively pushy. Trainees are better than trainers at spotting training opportunities: it is in their interest to do so, whereas trainers are often deeply engaged in service and so inevitably let some opportunities slip by unnoticed.

Two examples of pro-activity follow. In the first, a coach is pressing the trainee to take a more pro-active approach.

---

FIRST CASE REPORT ON PRO-ACTIVITY

Trainer: *How many hips have you done?*

Trainee: *None.*

Trainer: *None? You've seen a couple, assisted at several, did half of one under guidance. And nothing since then? OK. You're going to have to make it fairly clear to the Consultant that you want to do one. Say, 'Mr X, there's a hemi-arthroplasty later on. I've done half the operation under guidance and now I'd like to do the whole thing under your supervision.' He won't take that as being rude.*

Trainee: *Yes, well I tried that and it didn't work, did it?*

Trainer: *Right. Well, if somebody's away, identify that and get along to that list. Have a word with the trainer doing the list and say 'Do you mind if I do this one?' and explain why you think you're ready. There's often one on a Tuesday or a Wednesday, and your turn will come.*

**Later** . . . The trainee has just done his first dynamic hip screw (DHS) under the close supervision of the trainer. After a debriefing that follows the operation, the trainer advises the SHO how to get another learning opportunity and how to do so in a way that will increase his chances of obtaining one and getting the necessary support to aid his progression.

Trainer: *When you know there's a DHS on the trauma list, what you've got to do is say: 'I'd like to do that. I've done one before, and I'd like to do another one if I may.' Pick your time to do that: they come up often enough. Say to yourself, 'This morning my aim is to do a DHS.' I suggest you'd be better to have someone scrubbed in, but make sure they understand that you're doing it and you don't want them in the way unless there are any problems. At the beginning of the case, you've got to make it clear between you and the other person that their role is to stand by and help out if you get stuck. You'll ask for their help if you want it and they shouldn't elbow their way in. And you must say, 'I've done one before, I'm completely happy with all the steps of the operation but the bit I anticipate I may have difficulty with is getting the guide wire right to the centre of the head. I may need a bit of help with that and in fixing the plate onto the screw. Everything else I'm very happy with.' And then the person who's with you has a good grasp of what you're doing and where they can help you, and be ready to take over if that's necessary.*

---

In the second case, we see how, under the guidance of a coach, a trainee is led to become more pro-active.

## SECOND CASE REPORT ON PRO-ACTIVITY

Trainer: *It would be a good thing if you asked more to do some of the parts of operations that you think you can do and you would like to do.*

Trainee: *I don't think I could do that. I'm not that sort of a person. I'm a bit retiring in some ways. If you ask me to do something, I'll always do it, but it's different asking you. I'm not built that way.*

Trainer: *Well, I am rather a pushy person and I suppose I expect you to take the initiative sometimes.*

Trainee: *If I did ask you and then you said no I'd feel really put down, snubbed.*

**Some weeks later . . .** After further encouragement by the coach, the trainee has gained more confidence about being pro-active and talks in a different way about eliciting training in the firm to which he is moving.

Trainee: *I'll see what sort of cases we're getting on the list I'm with and if there's nothing for me, I might just say, after the first month, 'There's a case I haven't done today and the other trainee has already done one of those, so can I please do the trauma list today because I'm free? Do you mind?'*

Trainer: *What do you think about your level of pro-activity?*

Trainee: *There's lots of room for improvement. It's given me something to think about, actually. I'm more aware of it than I ever was and I really am going to work on being more pro-active.*

Trainer: *You are more pro-active, undoubtedly. In the last few weeks, asking to do a particular thing, or asking to see something or be shown something, led to you being taught in a way that wouldn't have happened if you hadn't started it off. When you asked [another trainer] a question or said you wanted to do something, I never saw you rebuffed.*

Trainee: *It is something to work on, but it's hard. It's just the way you're brought up. Just by being there, you expect to get taught, I'm consenting to being taught. But I see the roles are changing these days and pressure of time. You have to say to yourself that it's not just being there, it's actually saying, 'Let me have a go at this.'*

**Three months later...**
Interviewer: *Looking back, was the encouragement to be pro-active welcome? Did it influence you, d'you think?*

Trainee: *I think it was needed rather than welcome. Before I came here, I expected to pick up things. I expected it to be a senior-led thing, that I'd learn just being there. But he's really turned my thinking on its head now, because not only should I be there, but I should participate and where necessary, remind people — 'Look, I really am here, I want to be taught on this,' and ask them. I think about being pro-active all the time. It's a concept that's really sunk in.*

The most difficult task for the coach is to encourage pro-activity in trainees but without feeling that they are thereby committed to granting all requests. Some requests will and should be refused: it is the style of the refusal, not the refusal itself, that counts. If the refusal is done pleasantly with a clear reason and, wherever possible, with an assurance that the request may be granted at a later stage, trainees do not feel dented or diminished and so do not retreat from being pro-active and taking their share of responsibility for their OJT.

In summary, the effective coach:

- encourages trainees to be pro-active, especially those who seem diffident
- re-orientates the diffident and the excessively pro-active towards a more appropriate style and level of pro-activity
- creates the conditions under which such pro-activity will flourish
- ensures that appropriate pro-active behaviour pays off for the trainee
- inhibits or re-directs, without snubbing, pro-active behaviour that is inappropriate in content or timing
- sometimes refuses trainee requests for hand-on experience, but never humiliates
- tells trainees in what matters or on what occasions taking the initiative is not welcome
- accepts that a good trainee will be impatient to progress and so will be eager for more responsibility or hands-on experience.

This creates the partnership between coach and trainer for effective OJT.

## ACTION POINTS ON BEING PRO-ACTIVE

### TRAINEES
- be active in shaping your training and eliciting teaching from your coach(es)
- avoid the extremes of being too diffident and too pushy
- scan all service for opportunities for teaching and learning
- ask to do things, but make sure you're ready for the responsibility
- don't worry if some of your requests are refused
- suggest to your coach solutions to your problems — you learn more than simply asking for advice about what to do.

### TRAINERS
- encourage your trainees to be pro-active, as this helps them to take responsibility for their learning and to be well motivated
- discuss the issue of pro-activity openly with diffident trainees — they need to know that you want them to take more initiative
- if you refuse requests for hands-on experience, explain why.

# 6   HOW TO ASK QUESTIONS (1)

> Question asking is the royal road to knowledge and learning.
>
> Seymour Sarason, psychologist, 1993

## THIS SECTION:

- **shows why questioning is a key skill in coaching**
- **explains the forms and functions of questions**
- **focuses on questions that stimulate thinking and reasoning**
- **suggests how to develop your questioning skills**

Questioning is under-used as a technique in medical OJT and is a more subtle skill than many coaches realise. Training is better if there is more questioning and it is done more skilfully.

### FOR TRAINEES

This Section is largely for coaches on how to question you in a way that helps you to learn effectively. You should look through this Section to understand fully when some kinds of questioning can sometimes be challenging, even painful, for you if you are to be stretched to the full. Some advice on how you should question your coach is in Section 11.

What is a question? What's the point of asking questions? How and why do they contribute to learning?

Questions take different **forms** and serve different **functions** and have variable **value** for training. Consider how these three ideas work in practice.

There are two basic forms of question — closed and open.

**Closed questions** have a known and fixed answer which is clearly either right or wrong.

　*e.g. What does DVT stand for?*

**Open questions** have several possible or plausible answers or even no obvious or uncontentious answer at all.

31

*e.g. What prophylactic measures can be used to prevent post-operative DVT?*

Other questions can be answered simply by a 'yes' or 'no' and so are neither obviously open nor closed. If a yes or no is sufficient as a competent answer requiring no further justification or elaboration, then the question is **half-closed**.

*Question: Can subcutaneous heparin be used to prevent post-operative DVT?*
*Answer: Yes.*

If the response of yes or no is not an adequate answer and the questioner can reasonably expect some elaboration, then the question is **half-open**.

*Question: Is subcutaneous heparin the best prophylaxis against post-operative DVT?*
*Answer: Yes, because . . .*

Here are some examples of questions asked of trainees by trainers. Can you say which are open, closed, half-open and half-closed? Which have the greatest value in helping the trainee to learn?

- *What do we call this kind of fracture?*
- *Which muscle is this?*
- *Do you know how to grade oesophagitis?*
- *Does this angiogram show good distal run-off?*
- *Would you evacuate this haematoma?*
- *How does this barium enema help you?*
- *Why d'you think it won't heal?*
- *How could you tell if it's infected?*
- *What options are there for managing this?*
- *Under what circumstances would you do an emergency laparotomy?*
- *How do you decide whether to replace the glenoid or not?*

**Closed questions** require relatively lower order cognitive functioning, often simple recall. They are appropriate to aspects of surgical training, as when the trainer checks that trainees know the relevant anatomy during operations. Trainees may be reluctant to answer a closed question unless they are absolutely sure they know the right answer, for to give the wrong answer potentially invites ridicule or even the dreaded public humiliation. Admitting one does not know reveals one's ignorance. The best bet, especially when the question is being asked in a group of trainees, is to say nothing and hope somebody else takes the risk — so teaching and learning are hindered.

Most closed questions asked by trainers are **test questions**, the function of which is to uncover whether trainees have the relevant knowledge and can give a clear answer — 'I know and I want to know if you know'. The limitation of closed questions is that if a trainee provides the right answer, this informs the coach, which can be useful, but it does relatively little for the trainee. It may make the trainee feel good to be able to supply the answer, but no additional learning is taking place. If the answer is wrong, then many trainers respond by providing the right answer. This may help the trainee, but it may not change the faulty reasoning or knowledge that lies behind the wrong answer. Genuine learning means changing the underlying reasoning not just parroting an isolated right answer.

**Open questions** demand higher cognitive functions — processes of reasoning, judgement and decision making — and so contribute more to professional learning. Open questions are good in helping trainees develop problem solving skills.

In a series of closed questions, the trainer is doing most of the asking and telling and the trainee is (the trainer hopes) learning by listening. In a series of open questions, it is the trainee who does most of the talking in having to give a thought-through response to the questions. The trainer, by asking good questions, forces the trainee to think. The trainer then monitors each response with a view to asking further questions or making supportive comments that will help the trainee arrive at a sound solution or conclusion. Trainees may groan at open questions because of the work that has to be done to formulate an answer, but to the coach the groan is the sign that learning is probably taking place.

## Questioning style

The style of the question can also be very influential. For example, if the trainer poses the question in an aggressive manner, trainees may be so nervous about failing to get the right answer (to a closed question) or about exploring possibilities (to an open question) that no answer is attempted at all. Of course there are times when a question should be challenging, and trainees are more likely to respond if the question is put gently with an explicit statement that the question is a tough one. Coaches should push a trainee hard through questions, but the manner adopted should be carefully fitted to the character of the trainee and the nature of the occasion.

33

Being challenging does not require the coach to be aggressive or oppressive.

Coaches should always remember that trainees are far more conscious than the coach of the nature of the audience who are witnessing any response from trainees: no trainee likes to be made to look foolish or inappropriately ignorant before peers — or nurses and patients. Public humiliation is not a sound teaching technique.

> If somebody asks a stupid question, you can show them it's a stupid question without making them feel stupid. There aren't many stupid questions from trainees — or from patients. Either they don't know or they haven't thought it through. If they haven't thought it through, that could be as much your fault as theirs and if they ask a question which demonstrates they haven't thought it through, they're often the most interesting ones because you can develop some really useful teaching from it.
>
> Consultant

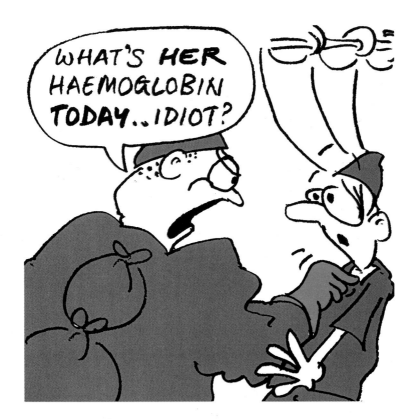

## Questioning to evoke higher order thinking and reasoning

In asking questions, the coach can have very different functions in mind — to get the trainee to hypothesize about possible causes; to speculate about effects; to reach a decision; to solve a problem. Asking open rather than closed questions can be more effective in getting the trainee to engage in the necessary, and sometimes painful, higher order thinking.

Examine these examples. Do the open questions stimulate higher order thinking more effectively?

---

### HIGHER ORDER QUESTIONS

1.  To get the trainee to identify and hypothesize about the character and causes of a condition
    - What's wrong with this patient? [Closed]
    - How has this condition come about in this patient? [Open]

2.  To get the trainee to identify and hypothesize about the effects and consequences of treatment
    - What does the book say the effects of this drug are? [Closed]
    - D'you realise what will happen if you do that? [Half-closed]
    - What would happen to the patient if you . . . ? [Open]

3.  To encourage trainee decision making
    - What's the right way to treat this? [Closed]
    - What are the options for managing this condition? [Open]

4.  To help the trainee with problem solving
    - Do you know how to solve this? [Half-closed]
    - Can you think of ways of solving this? [Half-open]
    - How might you get round that difficulty? [Open]

5.  To help the trainee to evaluate a decision or conclusion
    - Did you make the right decision? [Half-closed]
    - How will you know if that was a good decision? [Open]
    - What are the pros and cons of that? [Open]

---

A closed question is often answered quickly, since trainees either know or they don't. Silence usually means that nobody knows the answer. Open questions, because they demand much more thought, are often not answered quickly and silence often means simply that trainees are thinking. A glance at trainees' faces will usually indicate to the coach whether silence reflects thinking or bewilderment.

**35**

Trainers need to learn to leave a decent pause for this **thinking time** — at least 5 seconds. If the coach steps in too quickly — and most trainers do — thinking is interrupted and discouraged. It takes an effort for the coach to remain silent during this critical thinking time. Remember: the better the question, the longer the thinking time you should allow. The silence that follows a good question is hard for the trainer to tolerate, but not for the trainees.

Even so, a trainee sometimes comes up with a poor answer. The temptation on the coach may then be to step in with a correctional statement which provides a better answer. A more effective way of helping the trainee to learn is to ask another open question. This either helps the trainee towards a better answer or exposes the reasoning behind the poor answer. To correct the reasoning behind a faulty answer is better teaching than to correct the faulty answer itself.

Compare the following two exchanges between trainer and trainee. The first is short and snappy: the second takes much longer. Both cover the same topic. Is one a better piece of teaching than the other? What reasons can you suggest to defend your answer? Can another point of view be defended?

Exchange 1

Trainer  *Why do we catheterize patients with post-operative retention?*

Trainee  *To by-pass the blockage in outflow.*

Trainer  *No, there isn't a blockage usually. The bladder failure is a result of lack of muscle action, not a blockage.*

Now consider this longer exchange.

Exchange 2

Trainer  *Why do we catheterize patients with post-operative retention?*

Trainee  *To by-pass the blockage in outflow.*

Trainer  *Why should the patient have a block now when he didn't pre-operatively?*

Trainee  *The stress of the operation or the anaesthetic?*

Trainer  *How would that cause a blockage?*

Trainee *I'm not sure.*

Trainer *How does the bladder empty?*

Trainee *Well, the sphincter relaxes and the detrusor contracts.*

Trainer *Yes, so if there's no blockage, what could cause retention?*

Trainee *Failure of muscle contraction or relaxation . . .*

Trainer *Yes, and how might that occur?*

Trainee *Anaesthetic gases.*

Trainer *Yes, so why do we catheterize the patient?*

Trainee *To drain the urine whilst the bladder muscle is not functioning.*

Trainer *Yes, quite right.*

To develop your questioning skills, follow these four rules of thumb.

---

### FOUR RULES OF THUMB FOR QUESTIONING

- **Restrict closed questions to test questions**, they are appropriate when you want to know whether the trainee knows something factual.

- **Ask open questions in all other circumstances**, they are more likely to stimulate the higher order cognitive processes essential to learning beyond merely committing to memory.

- **Allow adequate thinking time** after an open question — at least 5 seconds.

- **Follow a poor answer with an open question**, it will lead the trainee to change direction or expose the faulty reasoning behind the wrong answer.

---

## Questions in semi-formal sessions

Learning how to question takes time. Fortunately, there are plenty of opportunities for practising the art. Most surgical departments have some form of daily meeting, often at the beginning or towards the end of the day, at which the consultants are briefed about their patients and/or recent admissions and management decisions are made. These are essentially business meetings, but are often and quite naturally

**37**

transformed into occasions for semi-formal teaching. In other words, for service reasons the trainer asks test questions to check trainee knowledge and then diverges from the real cases at hand to discuss wider issues arising from the case. Sometimes this is done in response to a question from the trainee. Questions are a natural part of semi-formal sessions.

Can the number of questions asked, either by coaches (whether Consultants or Specialist Registrars) or trainees, be increased to enhance OJT in these sessions?

In a typical, daily meeting of this kind, lasting for around 30 minutes, the trainer will, with no special or self-conscious intention, ask half a dozen questions which serve a teaching function. This adds up to 30 questions a week or 1,500 a year. Such a bank of questions is evidently a powerful teaching device. The questioning rate is around one question for every 5 minutes. If this rate can be doubled from six to 12 — an easy target to achieve if you try it for yourself — it means, another 1,500 questions a year. With a relatively small effort, the OJT element in a naturally occurring semi-formal occasion can be dramatically strengthened.

Of course the quality of the question is important too. Here are some guides to aid your practice. Do not try to use all four on any one occasion. Try one at a time. Once you feel comfortable with each, you will find yourself able to use more than one in a single OJT session.

## Ask one good question every time

One good question is more effective than a lot of poor ones — and saves time too. So if you know you're going to question trainees about a topic, ahead of time think up one really good question that will set them thinking, and make sure you use it. With practice, you'll find it easier to think up good questions on the spot.

## Practise one type of higher order question.

It's not easy to learn to ask, on a consistent basis, the open, higher order questions. So practise them one at a time. In one session, decide to focus on one type — questions about causes, or questions about effects and consequences, or questions about decision-making, and so on.

## Use the counter-question

In other words, respond to a question with a further question. *How shall I manage this patient?* asks the trainee. *What do you see as the options?* counters the coach. This makes the trainee think and informs the coach about the level and quality of the trainee's knowledge and thinking on the topic. It also gives the coach space to think about possible answers too.

## Nominate the trainee to answer

If you rely on volunteers to answer, some trainees will volunteer much more frequently than others. By sometimes nominating the person to answer you make sure those who are shy still get a fair share of the questions and an opportunity to participate. You also keep everyone on their toes. People tend to pay attention if they think there's a chance that they will be called on to answer.

## Role reversals — getting trainees to ask questions

Most question-and-answer sessions are trainer-led — the trainer asks the questions and the trainees provide (some of) the answers. As we have seen, there is a danger that the coach ends up asking mostly test questions, which do little to promote learning. It is the trainees who are sometimes best placed to know what they do not know or understand, so learning can be increased if roles can be reversed — trainees ask the questions and the coach answers.

Trainers often say they would like this to happen, but trainees don't seem keen to ask questions. Almost always this is because the coach has not used the best method for making trainees feel comfortable about asking questions.

Here is one approach that will discourage trainees from asking questions.

*OK. Any questions?* (One second pause). *Jolly good. Back to work!*

And so will these responses if a question is asked.

*If you'd been listening to what I've been saying, you'd know the answer to that.*

or

*Don't they teach anything at all in medical schools these days?*

**39**

Getting trainees to ask questions for their own sake is pointless. However trainees often do have questions but are nervous about asking them in case they end up looking stupid or inattentive or even ingratiating: most trainees' questions remain unanswered because they never get asked.

A good coach makes room for questions and invites trainees to fill the space provided. To encourage trainees to feel free to ask questions, try these alternative approaches.

> *OK. That was quite a difficult topic and I expect some of you have questions. Who'd like to ask the first one?* Count five seconds — only you will feel at all uncomfortable in the short silence — and if there's still no question, say: *Are there parts of what I said that seem at all unclear or difficult to follow that we might usefully go through?*

Trainees often take up such secondary invitations, because they have had sufficient space to think it out. If a question is asked, support the asking:

> *Mm. That's a good question. Now . . .*

or

> *I was hoping someone would raise that because . . .*

Sometimes a trainee will put a question in a very short and tentative form. By smart use of a counter-question, the coach gets the trainee to develop the question or move to an answer, thus making the trainee do more of the learning work. For example, try:

- **the counter-question for clarification** — *Good question. Do you mean . . .?* where the trainee did not mean that, and so talks further to clarify what was intended — which informs the coach about trainee thinking.
- **the counter-question for elaboration** — *That's interesting, but aren't you raising the issue of . . .?* which encourages the trainee to set the question in a wider context and make new connections.
- **the counter-question for role reversal** — *Good question : d'you want to make a stab at what an answer might be?* — trainees often know more than they think they know.

## ACTION POINTS ON QUESTIONING

- ask open questions whenever you can
- ask higher order questions whenever you can:
  - to hypothesise about the sources/causes of a condition
  - to hypothesise about the effects/consequences of a condition
  - to engage in problem-solving
  - to encourage decision making
  - to evaluate a conclusion or decision
- allow thinking time for open questions — 5 seconds — the better the question, the longer the thinking time needed
- ask challenging questions gently and slowly
- ask closed questions only to test trainee knowledge
- follow a poor answer with another question
- use questions to reveal and develop trainee reasoning
- get trainees to ask more of their own questions:
  - by allowing time for trainees to think out their questions
  - by making them feel comfortable about asking questions
  - by approving good questions
  - by asking counter-questions as your answer
- ask more questions in the semi-formal meetings you hold
- don't 'put down' a trainee who asks a question that seems stupid.

# 7 HOW TO ASK QUESTIONS (II)

> *Questioning is a far more difficult form of pedagogy for teachers than telling, because it is the least predictable.*
>
> Theodore Sizer, educationist, 1984

## THIS SECTION:

- **explains how to ask double questions**
- **explains how to turn closed into open sequences**
- **explains how to engage in holistic questioning**
- **explains how to reformulate why? questions**

These four skills are easy to explain but harder to put into practice.

## Asking double questions

When questioning, you may find it helps to ask double questions. In everyday situations we do not think about the question we want to ask, then take time to decide what its best form and function might be, and finally actually ask it. One common problem is realising that, after you have asked a question, its form is less than ideal. A way round this is to follow on with a second question which reformulates the first, thus making a double question.

You can double question in other circumstances too. For instance, when you get no reply from the trainee to your first question, reformulate it into a version more likely to elicit a response.

There are four common types of double question.

---

### I. REFORMULATE CLOSED TO OPEN

Here the coach asks a double question to get round the problem of having asked an initial closed question.

- *What's the way to treat this burn?* [Slight pause] *What options might we consider?*

Trainees tend to respond to the last version of a question, and in this case the reformulated open version is educationally preferable.

---

**43**

## 2. REFORMULATE OPEN TO CLOSED

This is useful when there is no response to the original open question and, for reasons of time pressure or the difficulty of the question, the coach wants a quick response.

- *What sort of energy is required to cause this cerebral contusion?* [Silence] *Is it high energy or low energy?*

- *What else can you say about this wound?* [Silence] *Is it granulating or infected?*

## 3. REFORMULATE FOR CLARIFICATION

The first question may be reformulated in a simpler or clearer form to help the trainees, who generally are unwilling to say they don't fully understand the question or see the point of it.

- *Do you think that's going to be stable?* [Pause] *Once we've got it back in place, d'you think it'll stay there?*

## 4. A NUDGING DOUBLE QUESTION

Another use of double questioning to support learning is to use the second question as a means of gently nudging trainees into a response. The second question may contain a clue or hint, which serves as 'scaffolding' to push trainee thinking and reasoning forward beyond what they think they know.

- *Why do you think we couldn't get it back into position?* [Pause] *We didn't push hard enough, or what?*

## Questions in sequence

The way we think about questions most of the time is that they occur naturally as one of a pair: a question is linked to, and is usually followed by, an answer.

In a teaching context, questions have a more complicated structure and usually occur as the first element in a triplet, not a pair. This is because the trainer asks the question; the trainee answers; and then the trainer has an extra turn in evaluating the answer. Consider the following exchanges.

Exchange 1

First speaker:        *What time is it?*
Second speaker: *One o'clock.*
First speaker:        *Yes, that's right. Well done!*

Exchange 2

First speaker:        *What time is it?*
Second speaker: *Two o'clock.*
First speaker:        *Thank you very much.*

If in everyday circumstances we asked somebody for the time, we would be astounded to be congratulated on our answer or have it corrected or be told it despite our ignorance (Exchange 1). This is because we assume the questioner is making an enquiry to which he or she does not already know the answer (Exchange 2).

The first triplet makes sense only if the first speaker is teaching the second speaker how to tell the time. In a teaching situation the participants assume that the teacher does know the answer to the question, and is asking the question not to obtain information but to test whether the trainee knows as well.

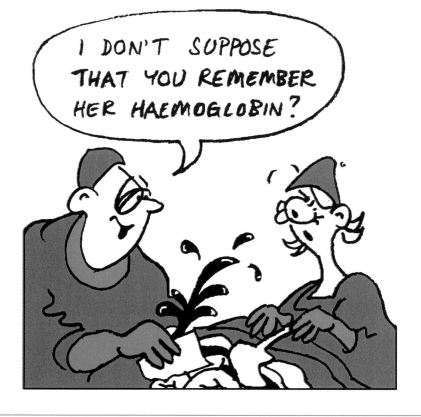

## Closed sequences

Questions with a clear, factual answer are usually closed questions, which often appear as the opening move in a triplet. At the end of the triplet, the trainer moves naturally to asking another closed question, so that the teaching takes the form of **closed triplets in a sequence**.

| | |
|---|---|
| Trainer: | *Closed question 1* |
| Trainee: | *Answer or statement of ignorance* |
| Trainer: | *Acceptance/correction/answer supplied* |

| | |
|---|---|
| Trainer: | *Closed question 2* |
| Trainee: | *Answer or statement of ignorance* |
| Trainer: | *Acceptance/correction/answer supplied* |

and so on.

There is nothing wrong with asking closed questions, but it is evident that the trainee is not doing much learning here but merely rehearsing existing knowledge for the benefit of the trainer. If the trainee gets most of the answers right, it is the trainer who does most of the learning — learning that the trainee is not very ignorant!

## Open sequences

More active trainee learning occurs when the coach turns a sequence into an open one. This is done by asking an open question, resulting in an open triplet of the following form.

| | |
|---|---|
| Coach: | *Question — open or closed* |
| Trainee: | *Answer* |
| Coach: | *Open question* |

Consider the following examples.

Open triplet example 1

| | |
|---|---|
| Coach: | *How should we manage this patient?* |
| Trainee: | *I don't know.* |
| Coach: | *What options d'you think there are?* |

The coach doesn't supply the missing answer, but by the open counter-question forces the trainee to think, which may reveal that the trainee has some inkling of what good management might be.

Open triplet example 2

| | |
|---|---|
| Coach: | *How should we manage this patient?* |
| Trainee: | *Operatively.* |
| Coach: | *Are there any circumstances where it might be appropriate to treat this fracture conservatively?* |

Here the coach avoids the premature 'closure' that is created by accepting or correcting the answer. Through another open question, the trainee is pressed to think out exceptions which will reveal the true extent of understanding. The trainee may finally be told that the first answer was 'right', but learning has been extended.

Turning closed triplets into open triplets is a relatively easy way of making the trainee learn and learn in a deep, rather than superficial, way.

Open triplet example 3

| | |
|---|---|
| Coach: | *How should we manage this patient?* |
| Trainee: | *Conservatively.* |
| Coach: | *What leads you to think that will work?* |

The coach declines the expected last turn of a closed triplet and neither accepts nor corrects the trainee's answer. The trainee is distracted from looking for a 'right or wrong' response and is pushed by the extra open question into setting the answer within the framework of a larger question. The trainer has initiated holistic questioning, each answer being logically related to other answers, which taken as a whole form a reasoned argument, in place of atomistic questioning or questions and answers only loosely related to one another with no coherent overall argument.

## Holistic *versus* atomistic questioning: an illustration

A 50 year old woman was driving on the motorway at 70 miles an hour. The car went off the motorway and flipped over several times. It took half an hour to cut the car into pieces and get her out. Surprisingly she was unharmed with nothing apparently to show for it except perhaps an acromio-clavicular dislocation. She was kept in hospital overnight for

**47**

observation. There was some discussion at the trauma meeting about how the patient's injury should be classified and managed. With respect to management, the decision was taken to do nothing — in the Consultant's words, 'leave it alone'.

The following discussion between the Consultant and trainee then took place, triggered by a seemingly minor question asked by the trainee.

| | | |
|---|---|---|
| 1. | Trainee | *So you just put it in a sling for 4 weeks?* |
| 2. | Coach | *What are you doing by putting it in a sling?* |
| 3. | Trainee | *Just resting the structures surrounding that injury.* |
| 4. | Coach | *So you're resting them. Why do you want to rest them?* |
| 5. | Trainee | *To try and encourage healing.* |
| 6. | Coach | *So which structures are you wanting to heal?* |
| 7. | Trainee | *The ligaments surrounding the injury.* |
| 8. | Coach | *So if the ligaments are under tension between the under-surface of the clavicle and the coracoid process and you tear them, what happens to the two ends of the ligament?* |
| 9. | Trainee | *They move apart.* |
| 10. | Coach | *How do they get back together again?* |
| 11. | Trainee | *[Silence]. They don't [mumbled]* |
| 12. | Coach | *They don't do that. They stay torn apart because it's a tight structure, and as soon as you tear it, the two parts go away from each other.* |
| 13. | Trainee | *[A textbook] says that it's best to put such arms in slings.* |
| 14. | Coach | *Logically, why are you doing it?* |
| 15. | Trainee | *To stop the arm pulling down and increasing the gap between the ends.* |
| 16. | Coach | *If the arm comes down, does it matter at all?* [pause] |
| 17. | Trainee | *Presumably not.* |
| 18. | Coach | *The ligaments aren't going to heal. So unless you keep them in a sling for ever to keep the shoulder up, it's going to drop down at some stage, isn't it? So why are you keeping it in a sling?* |
| 19. | Trainee | *To restrict movement.* |
| 20. | Coach | *Why do you want to restrict movement? [Silence]. Pain. You keep them in a sling for pain relief. And after a few weeks, when they're pain free, you get rid of it. If you think you're putting them in a sling for that to heal, I think you're being a little hopeful.* |
| 21. | Trainee | *You mean the ligaments will never heal?* |
| 22. | Coach | *Ligaments don't heal. In young children where there's a periosteal strip from the inferior surface of the clavicle, yes those do heal and new bone is laid down underneath it. But in adults those ligaments do not heal. So putting it in a sling's a waste of time if you're hoping for it to heal.* |

After the trainee's opening question, the Consultant could easily have said quite simply, 'No, that's not necessary,' and ended the conversation with appropriate service. Instead, he decides to make this a piece of teaching in which from the very beginning he sets himself the dual task of

- uncovering the faulty reasoning behind the trainee's belief that a sling is advisable in this case
- getting into place the correct reasoning by which the trainee would understand why the sling is not appropriate and for what reasons and so never repeat the error.

His first step, therefore, is to avoid giving a 'quick-fix' answer to the question (1) and so instead he offers a counter-question (2) to elicit from the trainee the reasoning behind the management suggestion. The answer (3) does not reveal the reasoning in full and so leads to a further question (4) from the Consultant. This proceeds over several moves until (11) when the trainee begins to see the flaw in his argument. The Consultant (12) spells this out in full.

At this point, however, the trainee comes back (13) with a defence of his preferred management option on the grounds that a book advises it. The coach ignores this diversionary appeal to authority and presses (14) for the logic behind the trainee's line of argument. This continues until at (20) the trainee has no answers left and falls silent. At (21) the penny has finally dropped that in this case the ligaments do not heal and so the sling is pointless. The coach concludes (22) by telling an exception to the generalisation implicit in the trainee's question.

This exchange took two and a quarter minutes. The trainee has, however, probably learned much. Through questioning, the faulty reasoning has been elicited, then subverted and finally replaced by correct reasoning. The nine questions asked by the coach are not nine isolated questions, but a holistic sequence held together by the governing intention to elicit and correct the trainee's reasoning, not his answer.

The consultant in this case offered the following comments.

> It's always a challenge for juniors to have to think why, to go through the steps of why they're doing what they do. The best way is not for me to give information, it's extracting from them and making them work through their thought processes, sorting through the problem, unless they come up with the answer in the end. This is better learning than just getting spoon-fed. If I asked closed questions, I'd just get standard one-word answers. In medicine, a lot of it is reasoning, thinking your way through the problem. I think open questions test people's reasoning more.

Holistic questioning is rare; it is a difficult skill to master, since there has to be self-control by the coach to avoid sliding into a simple telling of the correct answer. Practice is essential to keep an overall intention of eliciting faulty reasoning, getting the trainee to recognise why it is faulty, before working together to replace it — one hopes permanently — with the right reasoning.

There is, however, a danger in holistic questioning. Because the coach's questions are inter-connected, the trainee may find it difficult to see the purpose of the line of questioning, and so feel insecure or simply lose the thread. *I didn't know what he was driving at*, becomes the bewildered trainee's complaint. There are ways round this for the trainer, either as a prelude (*I need to talk you through this, so stick with me for a minute . . .*) or as a summary tail-piece (*That may have seemed a long way round, but perhaps you see now that . . .*). Trainees need to learn to trust trainers who use holistic questioning on a regular basis.

## Transforming why? questions from trainees

Eliciting the reasoning behind trainee thinking or action is often achieved by a coach through a why? question. Indeed, this is the most common way in which trainers demand explanations from trainees.

> *Why did you . . . ?*
> *Why would you . . . ?*
> *Why do you think . . . ?*
> *Why did that happen . . . ?*
> *Why is the patient . . . ?*
> *Why are you managing the patient like that?*

Why questions are easy to ask: whenever one does not understand, the obvious step is ask why? But why questions have two serious weaknesses:

- they can be very threatening to trainees, putting them immediately on the defensive, which inhibits deep thinking
- they are highly ambiguous.

And the ambiguity increases the sense of threat.

*Why?* can mean . . .

- what is your intention when you . . . ?
- what is your goal when you . . . ?
- what motivated you when you . . . ?
- what reason do you have for doing . . . ?
- what is the logical status of your thinking?
- what is the causal chain involved here?
- what processes are at work here?
- what effects do you hope to achieve?
- what consequences will follow?

Whilst the coach usually has a specific version of the why question in mind, this is buried inside the generality of the why, so the trainee has the double problem of trying to work out what the why really means and the answer to it.

The solution is simple: avoid why questions and be more specific about what you mean. However, it's not easy to get out of the habit of asking sloppy why questions. When you find yourself slipping into one, try the expedient of the **double question**. You hear yourself ask a why question, so immediately reformulate it in a more specific version.

---

REFORMULATED WHY QUESTIONS

*Why are you passing a nasogastric tube? What are you hoping to achieve by that?*

*Why are you putting the fracture in plaster? What is it about the injury that makes you think a plaster cast is good management?*

*Why are you giving a mannitol infusion? What benefits to the patient will accrue from this management?*

---

Another way in which the coach can learn to reformulate why questions is to ask trainees to clarify any why question they ask — which also has the advantage of making it more likely that any answer the coach gives will meet the trainee's intention in asking the question in the first place.

FURTHER ACTION POINTS ON QUESTIONING

- use double questions to help trainees to answer your questions
  - reformulate unintended closed questions as open ones
  - reformulate too difficult open questions as closed ones
  - reformulate to clarify a question
  - reformulate by hint or clue to 'scaffold' trainee learning
- avoid sequences of closed questions — break them by open questions
- practise the art of holistic questioning, but make sure that trainees see the point of a long sequence of questions and don't lose the thread
- take care with why? questions — reformulate to make the purpose behind your question as specific as you can.

# 8 HOW TO TELL AND EXPLAIN

> *The professional may find it difficult to admit that, although he knows he is successful, he does not know how to tell others how to behave equally effectively.*
> Chris Argyris & Donald Schön, educationists, 1974
>
> *It is invaluable for young trainees to see . . . into the mental processes of an experienced clinician.*
> Lord Walton, formerly President, Royal Society of Medicine, 1993

## THIS SECTION:

- **describes different kinds of telling**
- **shows how telling can be linked with questioning**
- **explains how to use questions to get feedback on telling.**

The common form of teaching is telling or explaining — what is often loosely called didactic teaching. A lecture is simply a formal and extended version of this method. Mini-versions of the lecture, **the lecturette**, are used by trainers on ward rounds and in theatre, but they rarely last for more than a few minutes.

More common, especially in theatre, is the making of **occasional comments** which

- describe what the trainer is doing
- explain why the trainer is doing it
- give background information to the description or explanation
- are relevant anecdotes, cautionary tales, jokes and funny stories.

Quite often these are random and have no obvious rationale. Effective trainers match the content and style of their comments quite closely to the needs and experience of the trainee. This is much harder to do than it sounds.

A very inexperienced trainee in theatre will benefit if the coach offers an overall view of the operation, and then gives a mixture of description and explanation from time to time to maintain the interest and attention of the trainee, who will otherwise soon become bored or continue to observe but without significant learning. At the end of the operation a brief overview of what has been achieved can also be helpful.

53

Experienced juniors may need little in the way of description and explanation, but will have their needs met if the coach invites them to ask questions whenever they want to. Asking the inexperienced to ask questions whenever they wish is poor strategy, for they either don't know what questions to ask and so keep silent and learn little, or they ask questions all the time, which is distracting.

Both trainers and trainees give explanations. Trainers usually offer explanations, either on their own initiative or in response to questions from trainees; but trainees usually only respond with explanations because the coach has asked for one.

A related but rarely used method is the **running commentary**, when the coach offers a continuous flow of description and explanation.

> Operations are very rarely done as something that is being actively taught by the Consultants. In most operations you learn the operation just by watching it being done. It's very rare for a Consultant to say, 'Today we are going to do such-and-such an operation and I'm going to tell you how to do it.' They don't usually talk much. Very few surgeons help you with a running commentary. They start sometimes, but they soon lose track. Sometimes they tell you to ask questions, but you can't keep interrupting when they're supposed to be concentrating. They don't want a little voice in their ear all the time asking stupid questions.
>
> Trainee
>
> There's nothing like it in my view, doing an operation and describing what you're doing at the same time. It's difficult to keep it going though, because you get interested in something and forget to keep talking about it. I sometimes get a Registrar to talk me through an operation. He should be able to do it. If I'm going to depend on him to teach an SHO, then he must be able to talk the SHO through it. So all the more reason why he should be able to talk me through it. Part of the reason we have the Registrar here is for him to teach others as well.
>
> Trainer

A few trainers who are highly experienced surgeons can do this, but most can sustain the commentary only for relatively short periods of time during those parts of the operation that are routine. In the more difficult parts, when the surgeon has to concentrate, a lapse into silence is natural — but for the experienced trainee this is the very moment when a commentary from the coach is particularly valuable.

Even rarer is the **thinking out loud** approach, where the coach makes no attempt to judge what the trainee needs by way of description or explanation, but simply tries to put into words the mind's content in a stream-of-consciousness style. This again is difficult to do in a sustained way for two main reasons: one's hands can do things more quickly than any verbal account of the action; and many of the things one does are so automatic that the knowledge of how to do it has become 'tacit' or below the level of ordinary consciousness. Despite these difficulties, 'thinking out loud' can be very helpful to trainees in giving insight into the way experienced surgeons approach their work. In particular it can give insights into the process of decision making and the factors that influence the decisions — something that is often obscured from the trainee relying exclusively on observation of the surgeon at work.

Specialist Registrars and newly appointed Consultants sometimes find it easier to think out loud because they have acquired the skill more recently and the knowledge has not yet become entirely tacit. If you find that you are good at giving the running commentary or thinking-out-loud — some people are, some are not — then you might try to encourage your trainees to do it too. It may help them to think about what they are doing and it may give you some insight into what and how they are thinking. But don't try to force trainees to do this if they are uncomfortable with it. And remember that many people find thinking-out-loud and the running commentary particularly onerous and distracting when they are concentrating very hard on something they find difficult to do.

## Telling with questioning — the didactic versus the socratic

Telling, especially describing and explaining, sometimes called the 'didactic' method, is often frowned upon as a teaching method, on the assumption that the so-called 'socratic' method of teaching-by-questioning is inherently superior. Yet the various forms of telling play a vital role in training, even though, unlike questioning, they do not always exert much pressure on the trainee to engage in active thinking. The best training talk is a careful blend of telling and questioning according to the circumstances.

Uninterrupted telling always risks a lapse of attention in the listening trainees — some of whom are skilled in the art of looking as if they are listening when they are not. Didactic talk provides the coach with very weak feedback on its impact on the trainee. Telling is easily 'chunked' or segmented by the insertion of questions at regular intervals. There are two types of question that are helpful here.

55

The first is the test question, discussed in the last Section, which is often a closed question serving to uncover or check the trainee's existing knowledge.

*Do you know about . . .?*
*Are you familiar with . . .?*
*Have I ever explained about . . .?*
*What is . . .?*

If you don't bother to ask, most trainees are reluctant to tell you that they do know or that you have already told them and so will politely listen to your redundant telling and explaining. At the same time a silence in response to *Do you know . . .?* and *Are you familiar with . . .?* types of question often masks a negative — the trainees don't like to acknowledge their ignorance. So a silent response may usefully be followed with a further test question along the lines of *Good, then you'll be able to tell me . . .* Often trainees then find themselves quite unable to tell the trainer about what they claimed they knew, so there is an opportunity for the trainer pleasantly to remind the trainees that ignorance is no crime, and that they should not be embarrassed about revealing it.

The second is the **check out question**, which checks out whether the trainee is understanding or following what you are telling.

*Is that clear?*
*Do you see that?*
*Are you following me?*
*OK?*

Such questions also have the useful effect of maintaining the listeners' attention to your talk.

A particularly effective sequence is the **explaining triad** which is a sequence of three moves as follows:

* test questions →
* explanation, interspersed with check out questions →
* more questions to test or to further trainee understanding.

In other words, the coach, instead of proceeding with a long piece of telling:

- first asks one or more **test questions** to ascertain the state of the trainee's knowledge or understanding, thus avoiding the danger of redundant telling;
- then, in the light of the gaps revealed, provides an explanation;
- uses regular **check out questions** designed to verify that the explanation is being followed, and also usefully chunks the telling into shorter segments;
- and concludes the sequences with **new or repeated test questions** — to verify that the trainee does indeed understand and/or to take the trainee's thinking or understanding further.

This explaining triad is a more effective teaching device than the pure didactic explanation alone, because it keeps the trainee actively participating rather than being a mere passive listener and provides feedback to the trainer on whether the explanation is being understood.

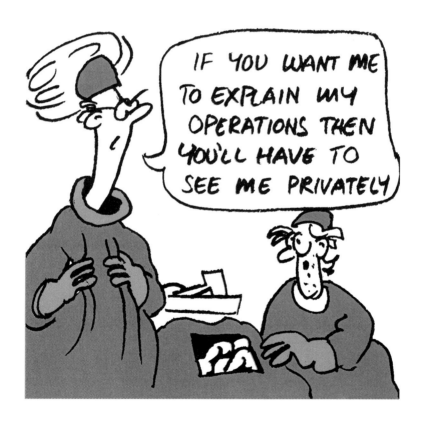

ACTION POINTS ON TELLING
AND EXPLAINING

- use test questions to verify trainee's current knowledge —
  making sure you don't cover ground unnecessarily
- 'chunk' telling by interspersing it with questions — don't just tell
- use regular check out questions to make sure that trainees are
  both listening and understanding
- learn how to use the explaining triad:
    test questions (to uncover state of trainee knowledge)
    explaining and check outs (to ensure trainee follows)
    test questions (to verify trainee understands fully)
- try spells of thinking out loud or the running commentary in
  theatre to help trainees
- if you can successfully model thinking out loud and the running
  commentary, then encourage trainees to try it — but don't force
  it on them.

# 9 HOW TO GET AND GIVE FEEDBACK

> *In my view, fair treatment of an individual means that he or she has every right to know, as closely as you can convey, what are the things that he or she can do better, and what is the best course to take for the man or woman concerned in order to further their own interests.*
>
> Sir John Harvey Jones, industrialist, 1994
>
> *All those involved in teaching can contribute by creating a positive educational environment, helping learners to achieve their goals by providing support and constructive feedback...They need to understand more about the need for, and ways of achieving, feedback, appraisal, openness and trust.*
>
> The Report of SCOPME, 1994
> (The Standing Committee on Postgraduate Medical Education)

## THIS SECTION:

- **illustrates the weakness of current feedback practices**
- **outlines the joint responsibilities of trainers and trainees**
- **illustrates good practices for both coach and trainee**
- **describes the dimensions of feedback**
- **explains the relationship between feedback and assessment**

Over a number of years, surveys have shown that lack of feedback is the most common complaint trainees make about their training. In many ways it is also the most serious, for feedback is essential to progression in learning. Bland reassurances are sometimes given, but this is not what trainees want.

### TRAINEE COMMENTS ON FEEDBACK

*He told me I was doing fine, that was it.*

*I don't feel I'm given enough information on where I stand.*

*What I would like is more feedback directly from the Consultants on a day-to-day basis.*

A lack of regular and clear feedback from the trainer condemns a trainee at best to learning by trial and error. No wonder, then, that trainees enter a desperate search for external feedback beyond their self-evaluation.

59

Trainees feel driven to indirect sources:

- inferring that all is going well if the Consultant doesn't complain
- picking up 'vibes'
- making comparisons with one's peers
- guessing at one's competence on the basis of how well one is coping.

These are useful but not reliable guides.

---

### INDIRECT SOURCES OF FEEDBACK: TRAINEE REPORTS

*You get feedback from Consultants either covertly or overtly. You do something, they're obviously very annoyed; you do something, they're obviously pleased. You learn to pick up the signals.*

*When the Consultant goes away, the things he leaves you to do on his list, that's a good indicator of how much he trusts you and lets you know where you stand.*

*The secretary's told me that one of the Consultants was quite impressed with me, but I haven't heard anything from the Consultant himself.*

*I think the Consultants feel formal feedback might in some ways detract from the system, the apprenticeship system, the traditional system.*

Unpublished 1994 Survey

---

Some trainees are reluctant to ask for direct feedback, for fear that it will be distressingly negative. Trainers are often embarrassed by the task and prefer to say as little as possible — though many seem to imagine that they give more and clearer feedback than their trainees believe. It is when both trainer and trainee back away from the task of giving and getting feedback that the trainee faces the greatest danger of inhibiting his learning progression.

---

*It's very easy to be negative about feedback and think that no feedback is bad feedback. Short of somebody sitting you down and saying you're doing fine, you're not going to be happy with what you're doing. It's not easy to go and ask people saying: "Am I alright?" Nobody likes doing that because they're worried what the answer might be.*

Trainee

---

We tend to think of feedback as a one-way communication, from trainer to trainee, and the responsibility for it as belonging to the trainer. This is a misconception. Feedback requires active work from both trainer and trainee.

The main responsibilities of the **trainer** in feedback are:

- always to be prepared to offer feedback
- to take the initiative in providing feedback
- to provide both positive feedback (e.g. what is being done well) and negative feedback (e.g. what is being done badly)
- to make the negative feedback highly specific and directed in a practical way to improvement, that is, it refers to concrete examples and is accompanied by advice or suggestion about how it can be done better in future.

The main responsibilities of the **trainee** in feedback are:

- always to be ready to receive feedback
- to take the initiative and ask for it if it is not offered
- to expect both positive and negative feedback
- to listen carefully to negative feedback, and to ask for some constructive, practical advice on how to remedy weaknesses or faults.

It is important that both coach and trainee treat the giving and the receiving of feedback as a crucial part of their relationship. For this reason they must do so from a very early stage in their relationship. If, sometimes with the best intentions, the trainer defers it for several weeks, then feedback becomes something the trainer would prefer to avoid and providing it is postponed yet again. As some trainees attest, it may then never be given at all. So trainees may have to ask for feedback. The trainee should give the coach some time to think about this, and so be ready to allow the coach some thinking time.

A golden rule for trainees is this: if you don't get feedback, ask for it.

---

EXAMPLE OF A GOOD PRACTICE

*Trainee to coach: I've been working with you for 3 weeks now, and I suppose you're beginning to get an idea of how I'm doing. I appreciate that you've been giving me some space to settle into your firm, but I'm now ready to hear what you think of my work and get advice on how I might make progress. Could we arrange a time when we might have a short, informal chat about this later in the week?*

---

**61**

Thus the trainee takes the initiative in introducing feedback-giving into the training relationship but in a way that leaves the trainer feeling comfortable about providing it.

Trainers should remember a very simple fact: most trainees are simply short of feedback and want more of it — but they do not feel they can say so to the trainer's face. A guide for trainers is this: praise in public but criticise in private. If trainers took the initiative and followed this simple precept, there would be a significant increase in trainee satisfaction with feedback.

> EXAMPLE OF A GOOD PRACTICE
>
> *Trainer to trainee: You've been in the firm for a week or two now, and I hope you're beginning to settle in. Perhaps it would be a good idea if we had a short private chat about your progress later in the week. Nothing too formal, more a sharing of thoughts. I can give you my first impressions of how you're doing. I expect you'd like me to tell you where you're doing well, but we can also talk about where you want to make progress next. How about Tuesday after clinic?*

Feedback clearly touches on the most sensitive and emotional aspects of the relationship between trainer and trainee, and both are often alert to every nuance of their talk in this sphere. This is why many trainers are uncomfortable with it and often eschew this responsibility. Giving clear indications of when milestones are passed and cushioning failure are not skills many trainers feel confident they possess.

Yet for trainees such feedback touches upon their key concern about success or failure in the job, and about whether they are making progress to the extent expected and at the proper rate.

It is one thing to make sure that there are opportunities for feedback to be provided: it is another to make sure that the style and content of such feedback make the exercise constructive, worthwhile and supportive of trainee learning.

Feedback is easier and more supportive of learning if the **coach**:

- gives it reasonably close to the relevant trainee behaviour
- bases it wherever possible on what has been directly observed
- provides positive feedback as often as possible — most trainees are starved of it

- avoids indiscriminate or vague positive feedback and focuses on something specific
- where criticism is involved, criticises the trainee's behaviour, not the trainee as a person
- offers clear positive advice on what to do, not just on what not to do, in future.

and if the **trainee**:

- tries to avoid being defensive. Trainees have generally been successful at school and university and find it hard after qualifying to find themselves making mistakes
- uses criticism as an occasion to seek detailed advice on how to get it right
- encourages the trainer to keep giving feedback — e.g. by saying 'thank you' for it — positive feedback will eventually come and be its own reward.

Feedback, then, is not a one-way process, but a commitment by both coach and trainee to co-operate in the most delicate but important aspect of training.

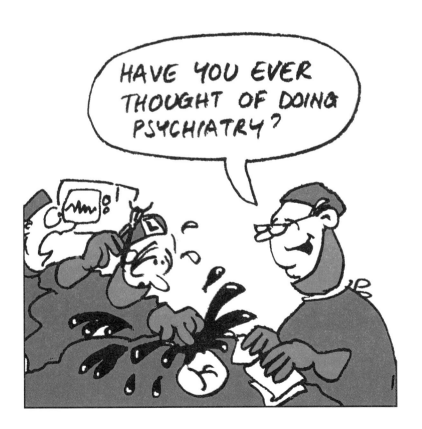

## Feedback and assessment

Many trainers are more comfortable with providing formal, summative assessments after several months on the job, whereas trainees also want informal and frequent formative feedback, integrated into OJT to guide their learning. Feedback and assessment are different but closely related concepts. They are often confused, so trainees are in danger of getting neither in any adequate form. Trainers and trainees need to clarify their thinking on the two concepts. The following set of antitheses helps.

---

### THE DIMENSIONS OF FEEDBACK AND ASSESSMENT

**Formal *versus* informal**
An official or formal assessment *versus* an informal feedback not intended to have official standing.

**Oral *versus* written**
Feedback is usually spoken and rarely written, whereas assessment may be spoken but often is put in writing, which may or may not be made available to the trainee.

**Immediate *versus* delayed**
Given during or directly after the performance of some action by a trainee *versus* postponed until some later stage. (Feedback may be immediate or delayed but assessment is normally delayed.)

**Direct *versus* indirect**
Provided personally by the coach to the trainee *versus* routed some other way — for example, a colleague reports to the trainee what the coach has said about him/her.

**Positive *versus* negative**
Praise or indication of approval *versus* criticism or indication of disapproval.

**'Formative' *versus* 'summative'**
Provided during a period of learning and intended to influence it *versus* provided as a terminal judgement at the end of a period of learning. (Feedback is formative more often than summative; assessment is more often summative than formative.)

**Unilateral *versus* bilateral**
Feedback and assessment from coach to trainee on quality of learning *versus* from trainee to coach on quality of teaching. (The unilateral approach is common. Where the coach introduces a bilateral element, the trainee is usually surprised and sometimes embarrassed.)

---

Trainees are looking for OJT feedback that is

- informal
- oral
- immediate
- direct
- formative
- unilateral from the trainer
- both positive and negative.

The regular provision of such feedback is essential to the learning that leads to progression — and it is the foundation on which a later assessment (formal, written, delayed, summative) rests.

## The feedback pyramid

The feedback pyramid consists of three layers, each being a different kind of feedback.

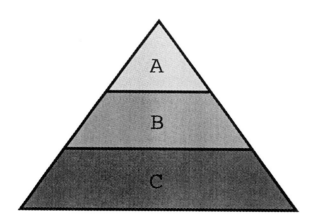

**A = formal and summative feedback in an assessment.**

There is a relatively small amount of this. If it occurs at all, it is provided by the coach in a rather formal way at the end of the period of training.

**65**

C=instant/short-term feedback on specific acts.

There is often a substantial amount of this form, both positive and negative, provided by the coach. The positive comes as the *Well done* or *That's good* and negative as *No* or *There's another way of doing that* when trainees are doing something wrong, inappropriate or dangerous.

B = holistic feedback on a sequence of acts.

It is this middle tier of the feedback pyramid — the feedback on a sequence of acts that belongs at the end of a coaching cycle — that is often missing and yet is a vital element in effective feedback.

> *When you've put a stitch in the wrong place, he'll tell you. What is hard to tell is how I'm doing overall. No-one will give you an overall judgement. Am I going to do all right in this specialty? Have I got the potential? Whatever your degree of self confidence is, it's still nice to be told. It's very hard: no-one will ever give you a straight answer.*
>
> Trainee
>
> *We have an immense responsibility to give feedback properly. Positive feedback is often very deficient. We Consultants just take it for granted. It's surprisingly rare for Consultants to say, 'You've operated well today' or 'You're making progress.' As a trainee you muddle along, thinking, 'Well, am I doing all right or am I not? If they're not telling me I'm doing badly then I must be doing all right.' I try to make a point of saying these things — 'You've done that well' and so on.*
>
> Consultant

A follow-up phase to a sequence of acts is the obvious way of providing the missing tier. This kind of feedback makes a huge contribution to learning and progression in that it:

- allows the coach to give feedback on the trainee's behaviour in the episode as a whole — holistic feedback
- allows the trainee to ask questions that might not have been possible or appropriate during service
- is retrospective in that it relates the feedback to the intentions made in the planning phase and also, if links are made with previous coaching cycles, potentially provides an evaluation of trainee progress

- is prospective in that it points forward to future learning needs and opportunities, thus feeding into later coaching cycles
- gives the coach an opportunity to offer advice/support.

This cannot be done all the time, of course. It needs, however, to be done regularly. OJT would be greatly improved if on some occasions on wards, in clinics and in theatre trainee surgeons were provided with feedback through an occasional follow-up session of a coaching cycle as the middle layer of the feedback pyramid.

Here are some suggestions to coaches on how to do it.

- **Let the trainee start the review**
  The trainee describes the good features of his/her performance. The coach may need to offer active encouragement here, since trainees are often unduly self-critical. The coach may need to add instances of what was done well.

- **Examine what might have been done better**
  Again the coach lets the trainee have the first shot at saying what he/she would have liked to do better or differently — and how and why. The coach then provides supportive advice through practical suggestions for improvement next time.

  Sometimes the trainee may be unaware of weaknesses or deficiencies or unwilling to acknowledge them openly. This is the most delicate part of a feedback dialogue. Through careful questioning the coach leads the trainee both to analyse the nature and extent of the problem and to probe possible solutions to it. Trainees do not mind being told of their weaknesses if this is done in an objective, matter-of-fact way that does not come across as a personal attack. Again, the coach is positive in giving advice on where to find the relevant knowledge or how and where to acquire the relevant skill.

- **Enthuse the trainee**
  Most trainees are anxious about how well they are doing and so may easily become disheartened. If trainees leave the feedback conversation feeling they have learnt something of worth and are looking forward to the occasion when they are confident their adjusted performance will be better, the coach can rest assured that the vital middle layer of the feedback pyramid is being provided.

**67**

## ACTION POINTS ON GIVING AND RECEIVING FEEDBACK

### TRAINERS

- give lots of feedback — trainees need it to learn
- remember how much trainees rely on indirect feedback — which may give quite the wrong impression of your actual views
- offer both positive and negative feedback — constructively
- be specific with the feedback — avoid vague praise or blame
- praise in public, criticise in private
- criticise the behaviour, not the person
- ask for some feedback on your coaching — it will help you get better at it and your asking shows that you think feedback is essential to sound learning and improvement.

### TRAINEES

- if you don't get much feedback, ask for some — be clear what you want and choose the moment when you ask for it.

### TRAINERS AND TRAINEES

- learn the different types of feedback — give or ask for:
  - instant feedback on a specific act
  - holistic feedback on a sequence of acts (e.g. over a half-day)
  - formal, summative assessment at the end of training.

# 10 HOW TO IMPLEMENT A TRAINING PLAN

> *Set targets which are impossible to achieve and you switch people off. Set targets which are too easy and you also switch them off. Set targets which are difficult but just achievable, and then ensure that you achieve them, and you will switch people on.*
>
> Sir John Harvey-Jones, industrialist, 1988
>
> *Educational supervisors can help by encouraging trainees to define their own educational objectives [and by] discussing and agreeing with trainees what should happen in order to meet these objectives, how this should be done, by whom, when and with what outcomes; in other words, to enter into an educational 'contract'.*
>
> The Report of SCOPME, 1994
> (The Standing Committee on Postgraduate Medical Education)

## THIS SECTION
- **explains why a training plan is essential**
- **illustrates how to construct a training plan**
- **shows how to use a training plan to support the process of training**

Some trainees feel that they drift through their training; it is not the guided journey they expected at the beginning. Some trainees learn from bitter experience that training should be planned and that the initiative may lie with them.

> *I learned hardly anything on that job. One thing I did learn is that you should start each job with an objective. That's one thing I've lacked. I think it's a good thing to start a job with a list of the things that you want to get out of that 6 months or 3 months. Then when you see the job coming to an end, you can say to the Consultant. 'I haven't done this yet and my time with you is coming to an end, so d'you think I could learn to do this before my time's up?' If you start with a list of objectives you can keep track of what you're learning and it will give you a bit more direction in your training.*
>
> Trainee

Apprenticeship-by-coaching is structured training that is planned and monitored and then adjusted in the light of experience. Giving direction and purpose to training is a difficult ideal to achieve during clinical practice and service unless the coach and the trainee co-operate to agree upon a training plan to guide the process of training.

**69**

A training plan is an agreement between coach and trainee on what is to be achieved in a given period. It takes into account the trainee's previous experience, current levels of knowledge and skill, and aspirations for learning. It reflects the coach's pattern of work and the expectations of what the trainee can reasonably be expected to achieve.

## What kind of training plan do coach and trainee want and need?

Every trainee is unique and comes to the attachment with a distinctive resource of experience, aptitudes and aspirations. The coach recognises that each trainee is hoping to gain from the attachment a unique combination of knowledge and skill, which has somehow to be fitted into what the coach sees as an adequate and relevant specialist training. The training agenda is therefore a mix of what each party brings to the training.

A training plan works well if what the trainer considers to be the appropriate content of training can be adapted, by agreement, to the learning needs of each particular trainee. The ideal plan is not a rigid, bureaucratic one permitting no variations and imposed by the trainer on all trainees: but is a personalised plan which takes account of the trainee's learning needs and wishes as well as the trainer's expectations and requirements. When coach and trainee have a hand in making such a plan, both have a stake in its success.

What is needed, in short, is a way of making each plan different but within a system that can achieve this quickly and efficiently without having to start from scratch each time the trainer gets a new trainee. The rest of the Section explains how this is done.

The form which a training plan takes and the way in which it is put together can vary enormously from individual to individual and from one surgical specialty to another. All the suggestions that follow are by way of illustration and should be adapted according to particular circumstances, needs and preferences.

**70**

## Designing a training plan

A training plan has four basic elements.

> ### THE FOUR ELEMENTS OF A TRAINING PLAN
>
> - List of topics to be covered during training
> - Target for each topic
> - Time-scale for achieving each target
> - Record of targets achieved

The **list of topics** to be covered is a mixture of knowledge and skills within the surgical specialty concerned, relevant to the particular trainee for the specific training period.

An SHO expects to see, and be involved in the management of, conditions within the specialty, but both trainee and coach also need to consider basic surgical skills, courses in preparation for examinations, and opportunities to learn about research.

In the case of a Specialist Registrar concentrating for a limited period on a sub-specialty, the topics may simply be a list of operations to be done and conditions to be seen and managed.

For more senior trainees the topic list will often be fairly predictable, as coach and trainee seek to achieve full coverage of the field; for more junior trainees the topics may well be broader and take into account the greater variety of career aspirations or uncertainties. Training in detailed operative techniques may be inappropriate if the trainee is not intending to remain within the specialty.

The **target for each topic** is specified at an agreed appropriate level in a chosen scale of progression. An example of a scale of progression is given in the Table on page 17. For a particular operation a trainee may already be at step 2 (assisting) and may aim over the period of the plan to reach step 5 (doing on his/her own). To achieve this, the progression through step 3 (the trainee does the operation with the coach as supervising assistant) and step 4 (the trainee does the operation alone but with the coach in the vicinity) needs to be planned. Trainee and coach may agree that there is nothing to be gained by further time in step 1 (observation) and that step 6 would be an unrealistic aim.

Such a training plan can take the following form.

| | ← | Scale of progression | | | | → |
|---|---|---|---|---|---|---|
| Topic list | Step 1 | Step 2 | Step 3 | Step 4 | Step 5 | Step 6 |
| An operation | | | | | | |
| | | | | | | |
| | | | | | | |
| | | | | | | |
| | | | | | | |
| | | | | | | |

Steps 1 and 6 have been closed or blocked out; the remaining steps are left open to indicate what remains as part of the plan. As time passes, the trainee inserts any appropriate notation (ticks, number of cases etc) into the open boxes as a record of the training experienced.

The **time-scale** for achieving each target is usually straightforward — the training period. A more sophisticated way is to use the boxes to mark a time-frame — for example, the first month for step 2, the second month for steps 3 and 4, and the third month for step 5.

Two real examples follow: a training plan for a Specialist Registrar for a 6-month attachment to a knee firm in orthopaedics, and one for a 6-month SHO attachment in general surgery. Though the plans look rather different, they follow the same basic principle. Indeed, they illustrate just how adaptable the scheme is, permitting considerable variation in the light of trainer and trainee needs and preferences.

In the Registrar's plan, the list of topics is closely limited to the major conditions of the specific sub-specialty. In the SHO plan, there is a broader range of topics.

## The Registrar's training plan

During the attachment, the Registrar is to cover the entire spectrum of care of patients with knee problems and this is reflected in the plan by target columns covering everything from reading about a condition to unsupervised operating. In this case the clinic and ward columns have been set up as:

Presentation:   Seeing new patients in clinic and learning how to elicit critical history and findings of examinations

Investigation:   Learning how to perform and interpret appropriate investigations

**72**

Management:   Understanding the options for treating the condition and learning to devise a rational plan for a specific patient

Follow-up:    Seeing patients in post-treatment review, learning about rehabilitation and outcome measures, and understanding the likely result of treatment.

## Example of Specialist Registrar Training programme. A knee surgery attachment during orthopaedic training

| | | | Clinic and ward | | | | Theatre | | |
|---|---|---|---|---|---|---|---|---|---|
| | Read | Tutorial | Presentation | Investigation | Management planning | Follow up | A | PA | P |
| Meniscal Injuries | | | | | | | | | |
| ACL tear | | | | | | | | | |
| PCL tear | | | | | | | | | |
| MCL injury | | | | | | | | | |
| LCL injury | | | | | | | | | |
| Tibial plateau fractures | | | | | | | | | |
| Distal femur fractures | | | | | | | | | |
| Osteochondral defects | | | | | | | | | |
| Patella instability | | | | | | | | | |
| Anterior knee pain | | | | | | | | | |
| Arthritis surgery | | | | | | | | | |
|   Early | | | | | | | | | |
|   Unicompartment | | | | | | | | | |
|   Multicompartment | | | | | | | | | |
| Revision knee replacement | | | | | | | | | |
| | | | | | | | | | |
| Knee anatomy | | | | | | | | | |
| Knee biomechanics | | | | | | | | | |
| | | | | | | | | | |
| Courses | Total knee replacement course<br>Advanced arthroscopy course | | | | | | | | |

A=Assisting the coach
PA=Primary surgeon assisted by the coach
P=Primary surgeon

73

# Example of SHO Training Plan — General Surgery

|  | Read | Tutorial | See | Assist | Do |
|---|---|---|---|---|---|
| **ELECTIVE SURGERY** | | | | | |
| **Upper gastrointestinal tract** | | | | | |
| Oesophagitis, strictures | | | | | |
| Peptic ulceration | | | | | |
| Crohn's disease | | | | | |
| Appendicitis | | | | | ! |
| Oesophageal, gastric neoplasms | | | | | |
| **Liver, biliary tract, pancreas and spleen** | | | | | |
| Jaundice | | | | | |
| Management of gallstones | | | ! | | |
| ERCP | | | ! | | |
| Cholecystectomy | | | ! | | |
| Pancreatitis | | | | | |
| Tumours | | | | | |
| Splenectomy | | | | | |
| **Lower intestinal tract** | | | | | |
| Ulcerative colitis | | | | | |
| Diverticulitis | | | | | |
| Colo-rectal tumours | | ! | | | |
| Haemorrhoids | | | | | |
| Ano-rectal sepsis/fissure | | | | | |
| Volvulus | | | | | |
| **Breast and endocrine Surgery** | | | | | |
| Benign breast disease | | | | | |
| Breast neoplasia | | ! | | | |
| Thyroid diseases | | | | | |
| Salivary glands | | | | | |
| Adrenal glands | | | | | |
| **Vascular surgery** | | | | | |
| Aortic aneurysm | | | | | |
| Varicose veins | | | | | ! |
| Carotid surgery | | | | | |
| Peripheral vascular surgery | | | | | |
| Amputation | | | | | |

**74**

|  | Read | Tutorial | See | Assist | Do |
|---|---|---|---|---|---|

**General**

|  | Read | Tutorial | See | Assist | Do |
|---|---|---|---|---|---|
| Groin hernias |  |  |  |  | ! |
| Acute GI bleeding |  |  |  |  |  |
| Acute abdomen |  |  | ! |  |  |
| Large bowel obstruction |  |  |  |  |  |
| Small bowel obstruction |  |  |  |  |  |
| Skin lumps |  |  |  |  |  |
| Examination of groin |  |  | ! |  | ! |
| Principles of laparoscopy | ! |  |  |  |  |

**TRAUMA**

|  | Read | Tutorial | See | Assist | Do |
|---|---|---|---|---|---|
| Head injury |  |  |  |  |  |
| Acute peripheral vascular injury |  |  |  |  |  |
| Blunt chest trauma |  |  |  |  |  |
| Resuscitation |  |  |  |  | ! |
| Management of abdominal trauma |  |  | ! |  |  |

**INVESTIGATIONS**

|  | Read | Tutorial | See | Assist | Do |
|---|---|---|---|---|---|
| Plain X-rays of the abdomen |  |  |  |  |  |
| Contrast X-rays |  |  |  |  |  |
| CT of the abdomen |  |  |  |  |  |
| Mammography |  |  | ! |  |  |
| Arteriography |  |  |  |  |  |
| Bloods — LFT, TFTs, U & E, ABG |  |  |  |  |  |
| Biopsies |  |  | ! |  |  |
| Ultrasound |  |  |  |  |  |
| Vascular laboratory |  |  |  |  |  |
| Ano-rectal physiology |  |  |  |  |  |
| Endoscopy |  |  |  |  |  |

**COURSES**

|  | Read | Tutorial | See | Assist | Do |
|---|---|---|---|---|---|
| ATLS |  |  |  |  |  |
| Basic surgical skills |  |  |  |  |  |
| FRCS course |  |  |  |  |  |
| Research and statistics principles |  |  |  |  |  |
| Basic science |  |  |  |  |  |
| STEP |  |  |  |  |  |

!=Priority topics/targets

**75**

## The SHO's training plan

The SHO's plan is less complex in its target steps — **read**, **tutorial**, **see**, **assist**, **do** can be applied to most of the chosen topics. This simplified set of targets matches the learning needs of the trainee, whose aim in the attachment is to gain some knowledge across the whole specialty rather than a more comprehensive coverage of a particular area. Inappropriate boxes have been closed. Arising out of discussion and agreement between coach and trainee, boxes have been closed either because the trainer thinks them unachievable or because the trainee thinks they will not be of value to his training at this point. To sharpen the plan, the notation '!' has been used to indicate those topics and targets which coach and trainee intend to make a priority in the first half of the attachment.

Every coach and trainee can thus use the system to meet their needs arising out of their specialty, local circumstances and personal situations. Further hints on planning are given in the account of the planning meeting described below.

## Using the training plan

The training plan is just a document unless it is used as a tool to give direction and coherence to the training process. The plan should be held by the trainee who keeps it to hand throughout the attachment. As a target is reached, this is checked on the plan. A pro-active trainee will steer training to those aspects of the plan that are in danger of being neglected or overlooked.

A conscientious coach may ask to look at the plan from time to time, partly to monitor progression and partly to remind themselves of what remains to be done.

A joint look at the plan is particularly useful when discussing a forthcoming operating list or clinic, so that the targets can influence the role the trainee is to adopt in relevant operations or examinations as a kind of training 'menu' for that occasion.

In this way the balance of training swings away from opportunistic and unplanned to planned and progressive OJT with minimal intrusion into service provision.

A training plan makes it easier for coach and trainee to talk about training. Short meetings linked to the plan provide continuity and progression throughout the training period. Coach and trainee naturally talk informally about both training and service as part of their daily work, but ideally coach and trainee need to meet rather more formally, in protected time, to construct the plan, to monitor progress, and then to evaluate whether the plan has been realised. Trainers and trainees normally have a meeting at the beginning and end of the attachment. The Section advises on how these meetings can, with the clearer structure provided by the plan, be of greater value to coach and trainee.

## Training meetings

We suggest three key training meetings.

---

TRAINING MEETINGS

Beginning      Introductory meeting
               Planning meeting
               (These initial meetings may be held as one session, but are
               probably better separated by a few days)

Middle         Progress meeting
               (Optional)

End            Evaluation meeting

---

These meetings should be planned by the coach in a quiet place in protected time for both. This takes effort on both sides, but the benefits are considerable.

## The introductory meeting

---

AGENDA FOR THE INITIAL MEETING

Trainee's background, experience, aspirations
Firm/team/department timetable
Trainee's responsibilities
Negotiation of a personalised plan

---

This is held as soon as possible and (like the other meetings) should last about 20 minutes. Though all can be done on a single occasion, it is best split into two shorter meetings.

**77**

Coach and trainee introduce themselves to 'break the ice'. The coach takes care to set the trainee at ease — he or she may well be apprehensive — since an honest and open relationship is a prerequisite for good training. The coach has the following initial agenda:

- ask the trainee to describe previous posts and experience (and so bring a CV to the meeting)
- ask the trainee about their career hopes, intentions and plans
- ask the trainee about examination record and intentions
- ask the trainee about recent relevant operating experience.

This encourages the trainee to make an early and active contribution to the discussion and demonstrates the coach's interest in the trainee. In the second part of the agenda the coach talks about

- the service commitment of the job
- the weekly time-table of work, including free time/study time
- what is expected of the trainee
- the people in the firm/team and department with whom the trainee will be working, including their routines and styles.

In the last part of the initial meeting, the coach describes the partnership aspect to the training and encourages a pro-active approach from the trainee. The concept of OJT and its relation to service delivery is explained.

It is easiest to explain the training plan by showing the trainee a draft copy, based on the experience of similar previous trainees. An experienced junior will be able to proceed to negotiating the plan there and then. Less experienced juniors, and those new to the hospital and/or specialty, will probably be too overloaded with new information to contribute properly. Such trainees should take the plan away for reflection and come to a further meeting a few days later to devise the plan.

In some cases it may be better to let the trainee settle in for a few weeks before constructing the training plan. This has the advantage that the trainee, now being more familiar with the specialty or sub-specialty and the routines of the department, is better placed to take a more active role in shaping the plan.

## The planning meeting

The coach and trainee discuss, negotiate and complete the plan. It is important at this stage to stress that the plan is not a standard document but is to be personalised through discussion. Modification, perhaps extensive, is the norm. The trainee may suggest changes to the topics and target steps, and which ones should be opened and closed. This is the first opportunity for the trainee to be pro-active and for the coach to show flexibility and responsiveness.

Once the plan has been agreed, the coach arranges for the final version to be typed up and returned to the trainee. If a master copy is kept on a computer, the personalised version can be produced easily and quickly.

79

## The progress meeting

---

### AGENDA FOR THE PROGRESS MEETING

Check progress
Record achievements
Identify missed targets
Modify the plan
Specify new targets

---

This is held at any mutually convenient time around the middle of the attachment. It should be held in a quiet place in protected time, since it is more formal than the chats which occur as part of the everyday coaching cycles and feedback sessions.

This meeting provides the opportunity for coach and trainee to:

- examine the extent to which the agreed plan has been executed
- check the extent of the trainee's progress in reaching the targets
- record where targets have been reached or exceeded
- analyse the reasons, if any aspects of the plan have fallen short
- revise the plan
- identify key topics or targets on which training should focus.

Where logistical or learning problems emerge, coach and trainee agree strategies to ensure that they are overcome within a modified plan.

This meeting may not be necessary if coach and trainee use the plan on a regular basis and both are confident that the implementation of the plan is being monitored and modified to meet the trainee's needs.

## The evaluation meeting

---

### AGENDA FOR THE EVALUATION MEETING

Review the plan
Offer summative assessment
Link to next attachment
Get feedback on coaching

---

This is held in the last few days of the post to conclude the training agreement and evaluate the effectiveness of the training plan and the achievements of the trainee.

This meeting will be of great significance to the trainee, since this is the occasion where the coach provides the summative feedback which serves as the formal assessment of trainee progress through the whole period of the attachment. There is positive feedback on the trainee's specific achievements in relation to the milestones of the specialty. New targets are outlined. In areas of relative weakness, the coach explores strategies for improvement which may well be carried forward into the next attachment.

It is not, however, just a one-way process, for the coach should invite the trainee to comment on the quality of training. If the relationship is open and positive, neither party need be embarrassed. Comments on those areas where the training has been particularly supportive, as well as on areas where more help might have been useful, make this meeting reciprocally valuable. The coach cannot expect to get better at coaching in the absence of a judicious mix of detailed positive and negative feedback from trainees.

## Are training plans practicable?

Most trainers accept that a written training plan is preferable to a conversation alone, but rightly point to the difficulty of finding the time for the meetings. If a Consultant is training just one Specialist Registrar for a period of a year or more, the time can be found. Difficulties arise when the Consultant has the responsibility for one or more SHOs as well, or for juniors who join the team for very short periods of just 2 or 3 months.

In these circumstances we believe that a Specialist Registrar, who has agreed a training plan for himself/herself with the Consultant, can be given delegated responsibility for constructing the plan with the SHOs and for conducting the relevant meetings. The final SHO plan should be approved by the Consultant, who needs to be aware of its content in order to contribute to that SHO's training.

In all cases trainees should be asked to monitor the implementation of the plan, which is designed to encourage them to see direction and purpose in the training and to take an active responsibility for it. Trainees should be ready, on appropriate

**81**

occasions, to inform other Consultants, who are not their educational supervisor, about the content of the plan when it is relevant to OJT being undertaken with that Consultant.

## Trainee evaluations of the plan in practice

### ONE TRAINEE WHO DID NOT HAVE A PLAN . . .

*I think it's actually good to have a structure. That's what's lacking, to be quite honest. I think it would have been better to have a structured set of goals, even if they were possibly unachievable. I think that's what the Educational Supervisor's role should be. Because technically we should have this Educational Supervisor who is a Consultant. He should sit down with us at the beginning of the job, discuss our initial goals, sit down with us in about 3 months and discuss how we're doing towards those goals and what route we should then take. Sit down at the end and we should have some feedback. I sat down at the beginning with [the Consultant] and he said 'Welcome' and asked us a bit about what we were doing. I never really had any targets. And I've had no feedback at the end. This is the way it goes. You have to organise yourself, really.*

### . . . AND THREE TRAINEES WHO HAD A PLAN . . .

*It was helpful the whole time. The other thing is that from [the trainer's] side, there is more interest in teaching me. There's a mutual awareness of the topics we've put into the plan. Previously, if I'd said 'Can I do this operation?' or 'Can we talk about this?' then sometimes the attitude was 'Well, yes, but not this time' or 'OK, but not just now' whereas with the plan, we'd agreed something, so I could always remind him that something was on the checklist and so there was more readiness to give me the experience so I could fill the checklist up. I was quite surprised by that, I didn't really expect it to work out that way. It definitely worked out better than I thought it would.*

*I thought at the time [the plan was made] that this was just another of those chats that would lead nowhere and make no difference, but I was wrong. It made me think about what I was doing and whether I was getting the training I wanted in this job. And I think it put a bit of pressure on [the trainer] to keep to the plan too. And I could always remind him about it tactfully — or even not so tactfully! In fact, I now want to specialise in [the trainer's specialty] which was not the case when I came here.*

*I think it was brilliant. It allows you to prepare, to get some more background knowledge to begin with, and that's a good point to start from. And then you always know where you are and what's going to happen. Then you can relate the different conditions together in the one compartment. Whereas doing it without a plan, haphazardly, you may not make the connections so easily. It also helped me see that my knowledge was improving. I could see by the end of my time in this firm that I really had learnt quite a lot. That's important to me, it's important to know that you do get something out of it. [My trainer and I] drew up a contract at the beginning, and we said we'd try to do these various things. We really did try to fulfil those, and if we saw an area I lacked, then he'd say, 'You know, you haven't done that yet, go ahead and do that.' And it made him understand my needs outside the firm, that I needed to go out to other [firms'] theatre sessions to see what they were doing. It made him more understanding of that side of things, rather than always expecting me to be present at my own firm's theatre sessions. Having a plan made me think about what I wanted and by telling [my trainer] and asking him the questions I needed to know, I suppose I guided him on what he needed to teach me on. That's the thing, I've learnt to try and set goals. Rather than just think about what you want to get out of it, try and set goals between you and whoever — the Consultant, the Registrar — and what you'd like to achieve in those, in the time you spend in the firm.*

ACTION POINTS ON DESIGNING AND
IMPLEMENTING A TRAINING PLAN

- make time for the meetings — it's worth the effort

- the first and last meetings (the welcome/planning and farewell/
  feedback) are the most important — your trainee takes them as
  an index of how much you value both training and the trainee

- the agenda for the **initial meeting**
    - trainee background, experience, aspirations
    - firm/team/department timetable
    - trainee's responsibilities
    - negotiation of a personalised training plan

- have a **mid-term discussion** to check progress and modify
  the plan

- the agenda for the final meeting
    - review the plan
    - offer summative assessment
    - link to the next attachment
    - get feedback on your coaching

- during the attachment, keep referring to the plan to steer and
  modify OJT — mid-course corrections are usually necessary

- encourage the trainee to record progression through OJT

- don't make the document (the plan) more important than the
  process of planning.

# II OJT IN THEATRE

> *I'm going to teach you how to swim just exactly one foot out of your depth.*
>
> Consultant Surgeon, 1996
>
> *The best performance is achieved by the combination of an objective a little further away than one thinks one can achieve with a relentless expectation from above that one will achieve it.*
>
> Sir John Harvey-Jones, industrialist, 1994

## THIS SECTION

- **explains why trainees need early operating experience**
- **shows how this can be done through planning**
- **illustrates how coaching cycles work in theatre**
- **shows trainees how to ask questions in theatre**
- **shows trainees how being pro-active in theatre gets results**

Learning to perform operations is central to the trainee's aspirations. So the provision of real opportunities for this by the coach is of paramount importance. Trainee surgeons who feel they are not wanted in theatre and who feel trapped on wards will be dissatisfied by their training and quickly show signs of low morale.

Consultants should remember that the greatest frustration of juniors is their conviction that they are not being given enough responsibility and that they are not being stretched. Rectifying this is the single most important action that the coach can do to improve the training of juniors. The courageous Consultant is willing to ask these two key questions of juniors:

*Are you being given enough responsibility?*

*Are you being stretched?*

If the answer is 'no' to one or both of these, then theatre is the setting where rectifying action is particularly important from the perspective of the junior.

Both coach and trainee should see every operating list as a training opportunity. Short lists relatively free of time constraints are obviously ideal for training, since this gives the coach more time for OJT that may be somewhat intrusive into service

85

delivery — for example, to demonstrate with an explanatory commentary, to encourage the trainee to ask questions and (most intrusive of all) to allow the trainee to do part of the operation. A long operating list in a limited time frame reduces the time for teaching, but does not remove it entirely, provided the coach is skilled in fusional OJT.

There are three ways in which the trainer can maximise the training opportunities in theatre.

- The coach teaches the trainee, as rapidly as possible, to reach steps 3 and 4 (See Section Four) for the simpler parts of the most common operations in the sub-specialty. By this means, the trainee is of practical use to the trainer in making service delivery very efficient and potentially releases more time for training. For this to happen, the trainer will need to ensure that the trainee is almost always in theatre for the operations and those parts of the operation which he or she is to master very quickly. This is the priority part of the training plan when it is initially agreed (see Section 10).

- To train the trainee as rapidly as possible means that the trainer has to give away as much operating as possible consistent with the capacity of the trainee to handle it. This is not easy, for the trainer can do the surgery better and faster. To do so whilst maintaining the interests of patients means having a very clear sense of the trainee's level of competence so that the task given to him or her is finely judged.

- The coach becomes skilled in fusional OJT, that is, has developed the skill of combining service with effective teaching in a way that prevents training becoming an obstacle to service delivery (see Section 2).

## Establishing the conditions for a training contract

Maximising training opportunities at the minimal cost of intruding into service is achieved when Consultant and Specialist Registrars commit themselves to a kind of contract in which the trainer agrees to be generous in giving away operating opportunities and the trainee in return promises to be proved trustworthy by seeking help whenever necessary.

The **giving away** element in the contract occurs when Consultants are willing to give away to their Specialist Registrars as much operating experience as they can

**86**

consistent with patient care. Since the Registrars are not then fighting for operating experience, they are not in competition with SHOs and can afford to be generous, cascading operating opportunities to them.

The **seeking help** element in the contract occurs when Specialist Registrars, conscious that they are being given operating opportunities close to the edge of their skills, must be ready to seek advice, help and intervention when it is needed and not wait for the Consultant to initiate it. But this will not happen unless Consultants take the lead in encouraging trainees to seek help — and the trainees believe that the Consultants expect to be taken at their word.

> In my first house job I was told by the consultant that I wasn't allowed to call him, I was only allowed to call the SHO. And the SHO was only allowed to call the Registrar. The Registrar could call the SR and the SR could only call the Consultant if the Queen Mother was run over in front of Casualty. That was one of the Consultants on my first day and he was serious. The Consultants here aren't at the end of the bed, but 24 hours a day, 7 days a week, they're on-call and if there's a problem with a patient, 'phone them. You wouldn't think twice about it. Four o'clock in the morning, you 'phone them and they don't mind.
>
> Consultant

> Every trainee goes through this period of being over-confident. You think you've got the basic skills, you think you're now acquiring some specialised skills. That's when you're most dangerous as a Registrar, you're going to do something stupid because you won't pick up the 'phone and say, 'Hey, this is what I think I should do in this situation. Is it the sensible way forward?' There can be an extraordinary level of confidence that inhibits one from seeking help when one needs to. So sometimes you have to be something of the fussing parent, to damp down this super-confidence. But then the trainee learns to make appropriate decisions and to call for help appropriately, and then you can back off and stop crowding them when they're desperate to fly on their own.
>
> Consultant

> [Juniors] must never feel afraid to pick up the 'phone and ask for advice and they must never be rebuffed by the next person in the chain. When they 'phone us, we're pleased to hear from them. We don't answer: Oh, what do you want now. It's not that, it's : 'Oh hi, what's the problem? Do you want me to come in?'
>
> Consultant

This attitude and practice then cascade down to the next level as Specialist Registrars, no longer having to fight for operating opportunities, encourage the same behaviour from SHOs in the firm.

How does this contract provide effective training with minimal loss to service?

87

Most trainees who are not quite sure what to do next in an operation are reluctant to stop and think, for this indicates to the trainer that help is needed. Trainees tend not to seek help unless they are desperate because they fear that, if they show they are not wholly competent, the trainer will give them fewer opportunities for operating experience. Trainees often keep on going while they have the chance until the trainer finally steps in. Knowing this is what happens, trainers watch trainees very closely for evidence of that rather purposeless busyness which indicates a surgeon losing direction. Then they step in uninvited in order to protect the patient and to avoid the loss of valuable time.

The contract gets round this. The trainer gives away generously on the understanding that the trainee will not waste time and pretend to a non-existent competence but will immediately call for advice, help or intervention when it is needed. It is a contract of trust. The trainee trusts that operating experience will be forthcoming; the coach trusts the trainee to ask for help. The coach trusts that if the trainee asks for a chance to operate, it will probably be a sensible request; the trainee knows that if the request is sensible, it will, if circumstances permit, be granted in whole or part. The contract has to be negotiated openly and explicitly by the trainer with the trainee.

## Planning rather than waiting for training opportunities

From the patients' point of view, undergoing surgery has three distinct phases — pre-operative, theatre, then a post-operative phase. There is a similar structure from the trainees' point of view, one parallel to the coaching cycle (see box p. 89).

As with coaching cycles, all three phases of theatre work are rarely undertaken on any one occasion. The important issue is that the functions of each phase are covered in some form at some time during the period of training.

### Before theatre — a planning phase

All the ways of maximising training opportunities rest upon the coach's skill in planning an operating list. This takes place before the operations, such as during the pre-op ward round where there is likely to be a discussion of the clinical circumstances of each operation on the list. As a last resort it may take place on

---

PHASES OF A COACHING CYCLE

**Planning phase** where coach and trainee decide the aspect of training on which to focus

**Service delivery phase** into which OJT is fused or blended

**Follow-up phase** where coach and trainee review the quality of trainee performance and any training provided and decide what to do in the next training cycle.

PHASES OF THEATRE

Before theatre = **planning phase**

Theatre itself = **service delivery phase with OJT**

After theatre = **follow-up phase**

---

arrival in theatre before the list begins, whilst scrubbing or even in the spaces between operations. Too frequent use of this 'last resort' approach means training opportunities are often missed.

Both trainer and trainee review the list for training opportunities. The aim is to devise a 'training menu' for the day, or in other words to reach an agreement on three things:

- which operations on the list are purely or largely service delivery
- which operations have significant opportunities for training
- which operations should make the session's 'training menu', that is, the ones which, in relation to the training plan, are to be the focus for teaching and learning.

The trainer obviously takes the lead here, but the trainee sometimes needs to be proactive in promoting the review itself or in negotiating the training opportunities.

This includes reminding the coach of the step level the trainee has reached, and aspires to, in each operation.

The trainee is then in a good position to undertake the necessary preparation to make best use of the training opportunity (e.g. by reading up the operation and

**89**

relevant anatomy the night before) and to arrange the work-load so that he or she is in theatre at the right time.

---

AN EXAMPLE OF PLANNING FOR TRAINING IN THEATRE

During the pre-op ward round for an orthopaedic list, the Consultant and Specialist Registrar agree that the first case, an arthroscopy of the knee, is well within the competence of the Registrar (step 5 — trainee does on his/her own) and will be done primarily as service delivery at the head of the list.

The second and third cases are total knee replacements (TKR), for which the Specialist Registrar is mainly in step 3 (trainee does under supervision) with some parts in step 5. They agree that the second case will be done with the Registrar as assistant, but with an opportunity for the Registrar to do under supervision the parts of the operation he still finds difficult. The third TKR will be done by the Registrar as principal operator, with the Consultant as assistant but ready to take over the most difficult parts if the Registrar feels he needs help.

The last case is an arthroscopic anterior cruciate ligament reconstruction, which the Registrar has not seen before. The Registrar will therefore assist and the Consultant will talk him through the operation.

Of the four operations only the third should slow down service delivery, which will matter little provided this is recognised in advance and the roles of each for the rest of the list are clarified to allow for this training opportunity. If time proves to be tight, they agree that the last case will be done with little commentary from the trainer, leaving the trainee in a mainly observational role.

---

Planning training opportunities is part of good coaching, but so is the skill of being alert to unexpected opportunities. For instance, when the coach encourages the trainee to ask questions whilst assisting, training takes place without affecting service delivery. If the coach in turn asks questions of the assisting trainee, this adds to learning as well as keeping the trainee from becoming bored or losing track of an operation that may be somewhat unfamiliar.

## Theatre — service delivery phase with OJT

It is not easy for trainees to ask questions in theatre, in part because so often, especially at SHO level, they are afraid of asking a question that will be thought by the trainer to be a 'stupid' one. There is an art to asking questions.

### TRAINEES — HOW TO ASK QUESTIONS IN THEATRE

This is not a matter of simply being enthusiastic and asking as many questions as one can think up. Rather it is a matter of choosing a good question and showing a sense of timing in when to pose it.

**Choosing a good question**

A good question is intelligent without a very obvious answer, but not one that is designed to be so penetrating that even the trainer is unlikely to know. It should show the trainer you are following the operation in close detail, rather than dreaming up some enquiry of marginal relevance to the case and it invites the trainer to explain what exactly is being done with what purpose in mind and for what reason.

**Timing it correctly**

Good timing is essential. Trainers do not give equal concentration to all parts of the operation. They are used to the more straightforward parts and so can do them almost on an automatic basis. The more difficult parts require very intense concentration. If you ask a question then, your question may be intrusive and so irritate the trainer. Or because it is intrusive, it may be ignored, which will make you feel bad. (The mask covering the trainer's face makes it hard to read when and how hard the trainer is concentrating.) So put your question when the trainer seems obviously very relaxed.

**If necessary, delay asking until later**

Sometimes you have a question but you don't ask it because you can see the coach is concentrating. By the time the coach looks relaxed, the operation has moved on. It can irritate the coach to be asked about something that is now clearly in the past and no longer in his attention. In such cases, wait until after the operation and then start, 'You know when . . .'

The coach should do everything possible to encourage trainees to ask questions and recognise the insecurity they feel about so doing.

Coach: *In theatre feel free to ask me questions, like 'Why are you doing it like this, tell me what you're doing?'*

Trainee: *Can I ask that during the operation or . . .?*

Coach: *Anytime. Any time at all. If we're far too busy to think about it, we'll tell you. Don't take that as a rebuff. Ask the same question a bit later, but most often, that's not the case.*

> Trainee: *That is a bit of a problem for me sometimes, if I feel I'm getting on somebody's nerves.*
>
> Coach: *If you get on my nerves, I'll tell you! I promise you. I don't beat around the bush, I'll tell you exactly what I think. So you feel free to keep asking anything you want.*

If the trainer is generous in offering hands-on experience to the trainee and/or the trainee has been sufficiently pro-active to obtain some, then there will be times when the trainee reaches the limit of his or her knowledge or skill and it will be appropriate for the coach to take over. Usually the coach watches the trainee very closely for those cues which indicate that the trainee needs help. Here is one coach explaining why he intervened.

> *I felt [the trainee] was struggling a little bit and I didn't know how to help him by guiding him without stepping in to find out myself exactly how best to deal with it. I felt he was having difficulty finding the next appropriate route. When you watch experienced surgeons at work, every single action has a purpose. Every time they move their hands to the instrument table, they pick up exactly what they want, do what they need to do, and then it goes down again. Nothing is wasted, no time is wasted — if they know what they're doing. But here the SHO was beginning to look rather vaguely at the instrument table, and then doing little things that didn't seem purposeful or trying things that weren't logical to me, so it was clear that he wasn't really sure how to tackle this part. I suspect that if I'd left him for a while he would have said, 'What do you think?'*

Trainees are often reluctant to ask the coach for guidance or — even more so — for the coach to take over. To do so is not, however, a sign of weakness, but an indication to the coach that one is aware of one's limitations and is always ready to ask for help. It is, then, a sign of strength rather than weakness for the coach can then trust the trainee in the knowledge that when needed help will be sought.

## After theatre — follow-up phase

Whenever possible, the coach should have a follow-up session to provide feedback (see Section 9). It does not matter if this is very short indeed, but trainees always want to know how well they performed. Simple praise is always welcome, provided that it is not done by formula and on appropriate occasions is supplemented by a more detailed talking through of how the operation went — identifying what went well and what might be improved in what way. Progression depends on a few moments of effective feedback.

Feedback at the end of a case is often overlooked for practical reasons — the trainer leaves theatre while the trainee closes; when the trainee has finished, the trainer is busy dictating the operation note; when both are having their coffee, other people are present and it's a bother to find a less public place for the more intimate talk. But with a little ingenuity, effective coaches do find moments for giving feedback — even if it is whilst scrubbing for the next case.

> Trainee: I think you get quite a lot of informal feedback during the operation. Sometimes it's very obvious like when they grab the instruments out of your hands and you know they're thinking 'This guy's a moron'. Sometimes we talk about it more while we're having a coffee if there's a wait between operations. But often the feedback's not really adequate, one needs to sit down more.
>
> Interviewer: I'd have thought a 5 minute de-brief at the end of the operation would be useful, on what you've done well and what you've not done so well.
>
> Trainee: I agree. That's something that surprises me in that it doesn't happen. You get the 'Oh, that's fine' and you get them grabbing the instruments as a clear sign that things aren't going well, but I can't honestly recall ever in my surgical career having 2 or 3 minutes with the Consultant along the lines of 'Yes, that was fine . . .' but then going into what could have been better.

The way trainers take over does sometimes seem brusque to trainees, who may not have insight into what trainers sometimes feel watching the inexperienced.

> ### TRAINERS OBSERVING TRAINEES OPERATING
>
> Watching a trainee struggle is frankly not at all easy. Most of us tend to get a bit impatient by grabbing the instruments, and juniors shouldn't necessarily take this as a rebuff — we naturally put patient care first.
>
> It's extremely stressful to stand and watch somebody muck a patient's tissues up. It's bad for the patient and it's bad for the outcome. Sometimes you just have to stop such trial and error learning. You graduate what you let the juniors do in all sorts of different ways, bearing the patient in mind all the time. You have to keep the patient in focus.

> We all enjoy operating and we all find it difficult, to a greater or lesser extent, to stand and watch someone doing something that you know you could do just that bit better yourself. It's a matter of discipline to stand there and keep your fingers still.
>
> If you're not sure whether the person opposite can really do something, you just have to do it yourself.

These are difficult matters for both trainer and trainee to talk about, but the lack of feedback may lead trainees to misunderstand the trainer's intentions for intervening and taking over an operation and to read the action as non-verbal, negative feedback. It probably lies with the trainer to take the initiative here and broach the matter. When coach and trainee can discuss the matter of such interventions without embarrassment on either side, the right partnership, especially in relation to feedback, has undoubtedly been established.

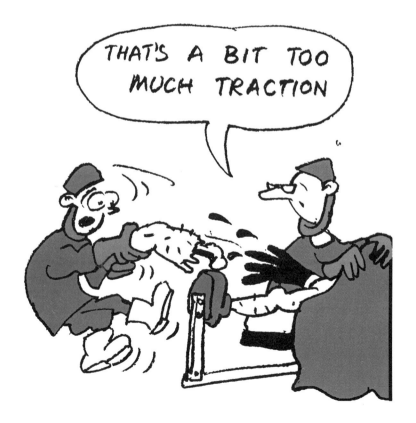

## THE CATCH 22 OF SURGICAL TRAINING . . . AND A WAY ROUND IT FOR TRAINEES

A trainer will more readily give operating opportunities to a trainee when the trainer is confident the trainee can operate competently. But since surgery cannot be learned through observation, how can the trainee ever get the experience to earn the trainer's confidence that he or she is competent enough to justify being given operating responsibility? Whilst operating skills cannot be learned through observation, the sequence of moves that make up the operation can be learned. A trainee who learns this sequence can then anticipate the trainer's next move and have the right instrument ready, move the retractor in the right way, etc. and so display to the trainer a familiarity with the operation that boosts trainer confidence in trainee competence and take the trainer to the stage where a request to do some of the operation is more likely to be granted.

*The Consultant had an attitude that when he was sure you had the confidence and knew exactly what you were doing when you assisted him — when he could see that you were anticipating his every move — he would give you some real operating to do under his supervision. I can see what he was getting at now, when I'm being assisted by various SHOs. Some of them know exactly what to do, how to follow you, how to know what you want next, you can see they're almost getting on to doing it themselves.*

Specialist Registrar

De-briefing is easier when there has been some planning — what is more natural for coach and trainee to check on the extent to which the plan was successfully executed? Planned training makes it easier for the trainee to be pro-active in asking for feedback when the coach forgets. It takes relatively little time to note any progression and to consider how any training objectives may need to be reviewed or revised.

95

## ACTION POINTS ON OJT IN THEATRE

### TRAINERS

- plan OJT into the theatre session — don't leave it all to chance

- work out a 'training menu' so that parts of the list have OJT

- if you can't plan a 'training menu' before the list starts, you can plan between or even during cases

- encourage trainees to ask you questions whilst you're operating if you don't mind this. If you do, make time for a few questions at the end of the operation

- provide specific feedback at the end of the operation or list

- use some of the coffee breaks or delays between cases for feedback or for training.

### TRAINEES

- play your part in devising a 'training menu' for the list — leaving it all to chance is too risky

- ask for help — it proves you don't exceed your ability

- anticipate all the moves and stages in the operations in which you assist — it shows you're ready for more responsibility

- learn the art of asking questions in theatre — the right question at the right time

- ask for specific feedback at the end of the operation or list

- you can use the more relaxed conversation in coffee breaks or between cases to learn something from your coach.

# 12 OJT IN CLINIC

> In the eighteenth century, there were only teaching clinics . . . The clinic was concerned only with the instruction . . . that is given by a master to his pupils.
> Michel Foucault, philosopher, 1963
>
> The guiding principle of education in the clinic must be that of flexibility.
> Donald A West & Arthur Kaufman, medical educators, 1981

## THIS SECTION
- **describes the four models of training in clinics**
- **shows how the models apply at different stages in training**
- **advises on how to get the best training out of clinic**

There is among surgeons an understandable concentration on theatre as the most important setting for OJT. This has led to an unjustified neglect of the clinic as a setting for training. In practice busy clinics are heavily oriented to service, but this does not remove all opportunities for OJT.

Clearly there could be better training if there were fewer patients or more Consultants. Better training may also be achieved through improved techniques of teaching and learning in clinic and the planning of training that is structured.

## Organising the clinic for learning

There are very many ways of organising a clinic: Consultants, nurses and managers all have preferred ways.

What are the main models of how clinics function and how training is fitted into the *modus operandi*?

For the clinic to run efficiently, three problems have to be solved:

- the filtering of patients to doctors: which patient sees which doctor — SHO, Specialist Registrar, Consultant.

**97**

- the achievement of a reasonable through-put (especially if the clinic is busy) and of reasonable waiting times for patients.
- the insertion of training into the above structure of service.

Four working models of the clinic are discussed.

## Model I — sitting in

Here the trainer (Consultant or Specialist Registrar) gets on with service delivery whilst the trainee (Specialist Registrar or SHO) observes. Whilst dealing with patients, the coach demonstrates, explains, asks questions of the trainee. In addition, the trainee may be sent from the consulting room or left in an examination room to deal with an aspect of management that is within his/her competence, subsequently resuming observation of the coach.

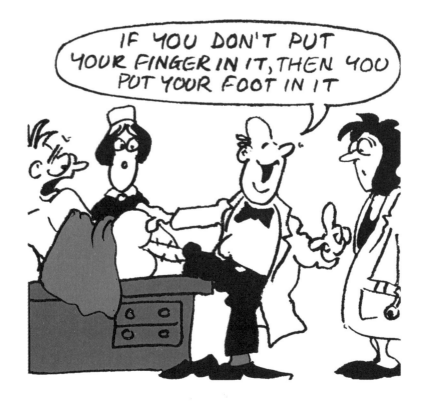

98

**Advantages** are:

- trainees may receive a considerable amount of teaching
- trainees see the full range of cases, including the rare or unusual, not just a filtered selection.

**Disadvantages** are:

- the trainee may lose concentration or get bored by just watching
- limited hands-on experience for the trainee
- the OJT is intrusive into service, so with just one doctor engaged in service the through-put of patients is slowed
- some trainers cannot afford this model because clinics are too busy, so coaching deteriorates to osmosis.

---

A positive report on sitting in

*For the first couple of times the Consultant let me sit in during the clinic. It was brilliant. The Consultant kept explaining things to the patients, but I think she was really explaining it to me, some of the time. I learned some really useful things, like the funny questions some patients ask and how to break some bad news in a gentle and caring way. I got some useful tips from listening to the Consultant dictating a letter to the GP. In between patients, the Consultant would talk about things that couldn't be said while the patient was in the room and she gave me a chance to ask questions, but the nurse kept giving us black looks because the queue was building up!*

Trainee

---

## Model 2 — service-led training

Here trainees see patients directly as a contribution to service. Patients may be filtered so that trainees see only new patients; or only follow-up patients, or any patient depending on their turn. Trainees deal with patients within their competence until they need advice, when they interrupt service to check up the line. The coach may also interrupt service, for example to invite the trainee to see an interesting or relevant case.

**99**

**Advantages** are:

- a high through-put of patients, since all doctors are engaged in service
- minor cases can be dealt with by trainees, to whom they may routinely be filtered.

**Disadvantages** are:

- a trainee may be excessively reluctant to seek advice from a coach, resulting in sub-standard service
- the trainee postpones the real decision, e.g. tells the patient to make another appointment in 3 months' time
- training is unplanned and in danger of containing an unstructured or random selection of cases
- trainees easily become restricted to simple or straightforward cases and their progression is thus limited
- rare or unusual cases may not be seen by trainees, unless called in by the coach to witness them
- advice-seeking potentially provides a significant opportunity for the coach to engage in training, but since the focus of attention is service delivery these opportunities are often left unexploited.

> If the coach decides to ask some questions and not just give advice...
>
> *When I joined this firm, I went to clinic and was told if I had any problems to get the advice of the Registrar. Well, I was new to the specialty, so at first I hardly knew anything and kept having to ask [the Registrar] what to do. He would tell me, but then he began asking me questions — what I thought about it, what I thought the options were, what I thought would happen if we did this, that or the other to the patient. I hated it at first, because I thought I was giving wrong answers or being made to look stupid for not knowing something obvious. I just wanted him to tell me what to do and then I could do it and get it over with. I realised it was helping me to learn and I did learn from him, but it wasn't easy. In the end, I learned that I could ask him questions and he told me lots of things. In my next job, I think I'll be more confident about asking questions once I've settled in.*

## Model 3 — service delivery with follow-up training

All doctors engage in service delivery (with or without the filtering of patients), but coach and/or trainee save up interesting cases, issues and questions for discussion during a planned or scheduled break or at the end of clinic.

**Advantages** are:

- no teaching during service, even when a trainee seeks advice from a coach, so the clinic is very efficient
- the teaching at the end of clinic can be open and relaxed, as no patients are present
- the trainee can, during clinic, construct an agenda of questions for the coach to answer and so be pro-active in shaping the training.

**Disadvantages** are:

- the training lacks structure and cases discussed at the end may be 'interesting' ones rather than those meeting trainee learning needs
- 'cold' teaching at the end of clinic is less effective than 'hot' teaching when trainees seek advice from the coach during service
- the post-clinic discussion is easily dropped or curtailed when the clinic is busy and so runs late, or when coach or trainee is tired or when either is called away to some other aspect of service commitment.

## Model 4 — planned training within service delivery

In this model, training is carefully planned. The trainee:

- contributes to service for those cases or aspects of management where the trainee has known competence and/or has been previously trained
- is given training by the coach on pre-selected topics where competence or experience is lacking.

The topics are pre-selected in accordance with the training plan to form a 'training menu' for this particular clinic. When either the trainer or the trainee sees a case

**101**

from the training menu, it serves as a 'trigger' for the two to meet to discuss the topic/case.

The 'training menu' topics should not be whole-case management of a particular disease or condition — this would take too long and be impractical — but a selected part of the management appropriate to the patient, e.g. if a new patient, the history or the relevant investigations; if a follow-up patient, the management options or rehabilitation or discharge.

The decision on the training menu is made just before clinic or in a follow-up session to a Model 3 clinic. The menu may not be adhered to in any rigid way — the particular circumstances (including which patients turn up for clinic) will entail making some changes, usually minor ones. At an early point in the attachment, the menu should consist of common and relatively simple cases, so that the trainee can quickly make a contribution to efficient service delivery. This creates space for more complex cases to be added to the menu and time for relevant teaching by the coach. In this way, the clinic becomes efficient and trainee progression is also achieved.

The trainee may see both new and follow-up patients, but the model requires some 'filtering' of patients. This may be done by trainer, trainee or nurses/managers, but requires clear understanding and careful organisation in the detailed arrangements that are made immediately prior to the clinic. With a little practice, and an awareness by all staff of the underlying rationale, this system runs smoothly.

**Advantages** are:

- the model supports trainee progression, as the filtered cases can change from week to week and increase steadily in difficulty
- the likelihood that trainees will see the range of cases specified in a training plan is increased
- teaching is highly focused, concentrated and less intrusive
- the trainee can seek advice from the coach on menu topics but, based on prior preparation, may then be expected to suggest options for management, including reasons for a preference in the case at hand
- the risk of insufficient time for follow-up discussion is avoided.

**Disadvantages** are:

- some preparation is needed and also has to be planned into the schedules of trainer and trainee
- the cases it is hoped will be seen by trainees may not in practice be available at the designated clinic or at a convenient time
- this model requires clear briefing of all clinic staff and meticulous organisation.

Note: much can depend on the clinic's physical layout. If consulting or examination rooms are distant from one another, it may be difficult for trainers and trainees to meet and talk without disrupting service delivery.

## The four models in action

Many clinics follow models 1–3 or some mixture of them. Model 1 is often used early in the trainee's experience and then dropped in favour of the preferred or regular model, which the trainer and the clinic staff regard as routine. Model 4 clinics are rare.

From a training point of view, the ideal model is a combination of models 3 and 4 , which mirrors the coaching cycle.

Phases of a coaching cycle

**Planning phase** where coach and trainee decide the aspect of training on which to focus

**Service delivery phase** into which OJT is fused or blended

**A follow-up phase** where coach and trainee review the quality of trainee performance and any training provided and decide what to do in the next training cycle.

Phases of clinic

Before clinic=**planning phase**

Clinic=**service delivery phase with OJT**

After clinic=**follow-up phase**

This may well not always be possible. To achieve sound training, however, any other model used as 'standard' has limitations. Different models are appropriate at different stages in the trainee's development.

## A mixed-model approach

It is difficult, on any one occasion, to provide in clinic a complete coaching cycle as occurs in the combined models 3 and 4. The advantage of the mixed model approach to organising training in clinic is that all elements of the cycle are indeed covered, but on separate occasions.

The mixed-model ideal achieves many advantages at the cost of the fewest overall disadvantages, but needs careful organisation and a full explanation to other staff of the reasons for varying the pattern of the clinic. Since nurses and managers are more interested in predictability and efficiency — using a constant method of getting through clinic in the shortest possible time — it is essential that the trainer explain the organisation of clinic as being both in the interests of such efficiency and in the interests of training the junior doctors.

An example of a mixed-model programme of training in clinic follows.

## Early stages

Model 1 (sitting-in) is adopted for one or two clinics, allowing the trainee to see the trainer at work, so that

* preferred practice is modelled by the coach
* the trainee sees the range of cases, including the less common and those of complex character
* the coach highlights the most common and relatively simple cases and what the trainee needs to do to prepare to take responsibility for dealing with them.

This is then immediately followed by model 4 (planned training with service delivery) with a focus on the most common and least complicated cases to achieve a rapid but high level of trainee competence with such cases. This has the effect of increasing trainee confidence in the work of the clinic and enhancing the part the trainee can play in service delivery and preparing the way for progression in training during later clinics.

## Middle stages

The topics on which training focuses are selected from the training plan (written at the beginning of training — see Section 10). It usually needs the trainee to show initiative in shaping a training menu: the trainee keeps an eye on whether the targets in the plan are being achieved and moulds the training process accordingly.

Either model 3 (service delivery with follow-up training) or model 4 (planned training with service delivery) or a combination are used to allow a focus on those cases necessary to a stepped progression in training. The choice of model may depend on the circumstances and trainee needs. As examples, if coach or trainee needs to leave early, model 3 becomes inappropriate; but if the trainee needs experience of particular cases to match the training plan, model 4 is appropriate.

At the end of each week or clinic, the trainee should keep a log of the extent to which the training plan is being achieved. If the plan has been well designed, this should take no more than a few minutes. This activity should help the trainee to plan the menu of topics for the next clinic. Gaps and omissions, once identified, become the basis for making minor changes to the clinic procedure to provide the necessary training opportunity.

An occasional clinic along the lines of model 3 can be particularly valuable in providing coach and trainee with a convenient opportunity to monitor progress with the training plan and decide on any action needed to ensure its continuing implementation.

## Late stages

At this point the trainee's learning is focused on the less common and more complex conditions. As the trainee has now no sense of being a hindrance to service and feels confident that any interruptions of service to seek advice will not be treated as foolish, model 2 (service-led training) can be used for much of the time. The trainee has a reasonable range of competence, so interruptions of the trainer are likely to be relatively few — thus maximising service delivery — but highly purposeful and rich in training value when they do occur.

At any clinic there are questions that trainers and trainees can usefully bear in mind.

Aide-mémoire for coaches in clinic

for each case

- is this on the training menu for today?

- if so, what action might I usefully take?

  - pass the patient over to the trainee

  - supervise the trainee managing the patient

  - invite the trainee in to observe my demonstration of sound examination, investigation, management etc.

  - keep notes on desk for discussion in post-clinic follow-up, especially where issues are most easily discussed in the absence of a patient — e.g. defence litigation, compensation, family circumstance, sensitive prognosis, etc.

Aide-mémoire for trainees in clinic

- have I made out my training menu for today?

- is it my own or has it been agreed with my coach?

- which way of organising the clinic is (i) appropriate to meeting my training needs (ii) practicable and convenient to all affected by it?

- before seeking advice from the coach, have I thought ahead and worked out the options or possible answers so that I can

  - demonstrate that I have given some thought to the matter before going for advice?
  - check whether I had worked the answer out for myself?
  - understand better why I was mistaken when my answer proves to be off beam?
  - ask the coach a sensible question to improve my understanding and reasoning?

Remember that you learn more if you allow the coach to approve or correct your thinking than if you simply ask '*What do I do with . . . ?*' to get his/her advice on what to do.

## ACTION POINTS ON OJT IN CLINIC

- before or at the beginning of clinic choose a clinic model:
  model 1 — sitting in (no service role for trainee)
  model 2 — service-led training
  model 3 — service delivery with follow-up training
  model 4 — planned training within service delivery
  and make sure everybody knows which model you have chosen
  for what reasons

- apply the appropriate clinic model to match the trainee's learning needs and point of progress to the circumstances and pressures prevailing at the time

- always use a 'training menu' to ensure that the trainee gets OJT
  from some part of the clinic

- give your trainees a copy of the aide-mémoire for trainees in
  clinic so that they take more responsibility for their learning

- keep nurses and other staff informed as to the purpose of variations in your adopted models for clinic

- make sure staff understand how, in the long term, variation in
  the clinic model speeds up service.

# 13 OJT ON THE WARD

> *Sir Lancelot strode across the ward, drew up sharply, and looked over the patients in the two rows of beds, sniffing the air like a dog picking up a scent. He thundered over to the bedside of a small, nervous man in the corner. The firm immediately re-arranged itself, like a smart platoon at drill. The Chief towered on the right of the patient's head; Sister stood opposite, her nurses squeezed behind her; the students surrounded the foot and sides of the bed like a screen; and the registrar and houseman stood beyond them, at a distance indicating that they were no longer in need of any instruction in surgery.*
>
> Richard Gordon, medical humorist, 1952

## THIS SECTION

- **shows how to implement a coaching cycle on ward rounds**
- **describes four types of ward round**
- **relates the four types to the achievement of training goals**
- **explains the three-minute round-up**

The teaching ward round is a hallowed tradition of the teaching hospital and images of it — not least James Robertson Justice as Sir Lancelot Spratt — are locked in the collective memory of surgeons.

Such a ward round offers many opportunities for a wide range of teaching techniques — modelling, demonstrating, explaining, asking questions — over many basic topics, both clinical and administrative.

**Clinical**

- presentation
- history
- signs and symptoms, diagnosis
- planning and interpretation of investigations
- patient preparation
- instructions for ward staff
- pre-operative planning
- post-operative monitoring, detection of complications
- planning rehabilitation

**109**

## Administrative

- dealing with relatives
- consent
- support services (social and community)
- discharge
- management of the firm/team

The ward is a favourable setting where **generic communication and social skills** may be modelled, taught and practised, including the following:

- establishing rapport with patients
- developing the art of listening
- obtaining accurate information in history taking
- eliciting fears and anxieties (declared or undeclared)
- interpreting non-verbal behaviour (e.g. facial expression, body position)
- using appropriate non-verbal behaviour (e.g. seating position)
- responding to concerns and worries
- explaining investigations and procedures
- explaining a diagnosis and its implications
- discussing treatment options
- breaking bad news
- checking that one is being understood.

In addition, patients will usually fall into one of four categories — pre-operative, immediately post-operative, late post-operative and non-operative, each of which offers different learning opportunities for trainees.

In many surgical departments, the formal ward round, whether business or teaching, at a fixed time and the Consultant accompanied by junior doctors, the ward sister, nurses and para-medical staff, appears to be in decline. Many Consultants prefer to do a far less formal ward round, usually with a junior, at a convenient time, often shortly before a theatre list and shortly after one.

The distinction between business and teaching ward rounds is a blurred one: teaching ward rounds often contain very little teaching and business ward rounds are potentially rich in opportunities for fusional OJT. In short, all ward rounds, whatever their designated purpose, whether they are formal or informal, long or short, should be treated as occasions when teaching and learning could and should take place.

Ward rounds potentially have a structure parallel to that of the coaching cycle.

Phases of a coaching cycle

**Planning phase** where coach and trainee decide the aspect of training on which to focus

**Service delivery phase** into which OJT is fused or blended

**Follow-up phase** where coach and trainee review the quality of trainee performance and any training provided and decide what to do in the next training cycle.

Phases of a ward round

Before the ward round = **planning phase**

The ward round itself = **service delivery phase with OJT**

After the ward round = **follow-up phase**

As with coaching cycles, all three phases of the ward round are rarely undertaken on any one occasion. The important issue is that the functions of each phase are covered in some form at some time during the period of training.

## Before the ward round — planning phase (for both training and service delivery)

This phase — seen by many trainees as the key to ward round training — is best done in an office or side-room on the ward. The trainee presents the Consultant and the others (other junior doctors, nurses, paramedical staff) with an update on each patient in turn. The coach offers explanations and asks questions of trainees and then gives all the trainees present an opportunity to ask questions.

III

The fact that the patient is not present allows

- a full and frank discussion of the case and the patient's condition and circumstances, including personality and character as it affects management
- questioning by the trainer, with the trainees being able to offer answers in private without embarrassment
- open correction by the trainer of unwise or erroneous answers and suggestions from trainees
- a debate on the advantages and disadvantages of various management and operative options
- an analysis of the degree of success of an operation and its effects and consequences
- a comparison by the Consultant with other similar cases, either currently on the ward or from the past
- a decision on the next steps in the management of the patient, after discussion of all the options and their merits
- a discussion on what needs to be done in relation to each patient on the ward round itself
- a selection of particular cases or patients or topics from the training plan that are a focus for teaching and learning on this occasion.

Each of these is an opportunity for teaching and learning.

During the planning phase, there is an opportunity for the trainer to devise, in discussion with the trainee, a suitable 'training menu' for the round, that is, from all the cases on offer in the ward, a selection that is immediately relevant to the trainee's learning needs and progression in the training plan. This usefully focuses both teaching and learning and certainly makes it easier for coach and trainee to raise questions about these patients.

If there is no opportunity to negotiate a training menu for the day, trainees can be encouraged to create one for themselves: a selective focus on a limited number of cases usually makes for better learning than more diffuse attention on every patient.

## The ward round — (mainly) service delivery phase

If there has been a planning phase, the round itself may be relatively short. Much of the time will be taken up in reaffirming the relationship between patient and the Consultant (and other members of the firm or team) — offering reassurance, boosting confidence and morale, providing information and checking that the patient has no outstanding problems, questions or complaints.

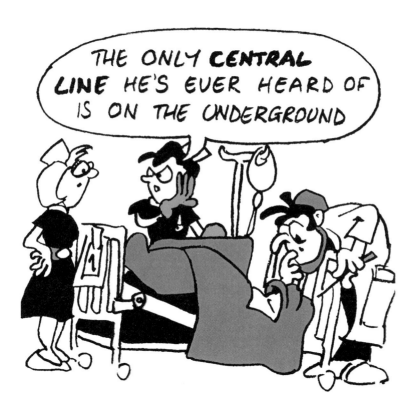

Any action decided in the planning phase — such as a physical examination or a check on patient mobility — flows naturally. Other topics that may be taken from the plan, such as communication skills, can be modelled by the trainer or undertaken by the trainee. Some aspects of training are best achieved if the trainee leads the ward round, with the trainer supporting, advising and de-briefing at the end.

As the firm or team moves between beds or rooms, the coach makes any additional comments and trainees ask questions that have sprung to mind from bedside observation.

If there has been no planning phase, the round takes much longer and the coach needs to be alert to the danger that the business aspect of the round will squeeze out the training aspect.

Trainees may be reluctant to ask questions in front of patients if they think that asking a question will undermine the confidence that patients have, and want, in their competence. For the same reason, they may not be responsive to questions from the trainer if an answer is likely to expose their ignorance or, even worse, errors of some kind. From the point of view of the trainee, questions on a ward round always carry the risk of leading to public humiliation. For this reason the effective coach develops a practice of encouraging trainees to feel free to save up questions for after the ward round.

## After the ward round — (mainly training) follow-up phase

The firm or team retires to an office or side-room, preferably where there is comfortable seating and refreshments. The team then discuss the issues arising from the ward round.

If there has been a planning phase, this final session will be short, as the business is mainly a matter of confirming the soundness of decisions drafted in the planning phase or changing them in the light of evidence emerging during the round.

If there has been no planning phase, the session will be longer, as there is an opportunity to engage in discussion of the topics and issues noted above.

## Types of ward round and their teaching potential

In spite of the usual distinction between teaching and business ward rounds, it is fruitful to see ward rounds as being of four types.

> ## TYPES OF WARD ROUND
>
> Type 1 — ward round only (teaching or business)
> Type 2 — planning phase and ward round
> Type 3 — ward round and follow-up phase
> Type 4 — planning phase and ward round and follow-up phase.

Type 4 is very rare but has the richest teaching potential.

Type 1 is very common but has the least teaching potential.

Types 2 and 3 strike a good balance between the need to use time efficiently and the need to use the ward round as a vehicle for training.

Some trainers use either type 2 or type 3 as standard, but each has different strengths and using them in combination is both possible and beneficial. Type 2 is particularly useful when the trainees are new and/or relatively inexperienced, since the open discussion before the round supports rapid learning. Type 3 is useful as trainees acquire more experience and familiarity with the specialty and with the Consultant — and type 3 is useful when time is pressing, since the follow-up can, under pressure, be brief.

It is common practice to make a distinction between a business ward round and a teaching ward round. The distinction is probably unhelpful, for it implies — in our view quite falsely — that some rounds are, and should be, teaching-free. This is neither true, for there will be teaching and learning on any ward round, nor desirable, for the art of fusional OJT is blending some teaching and learning into service delivery. In other words, all ward rounds are teaching rounds: but there is a sliding scale, with at one extreme some ward rounds having relatively little explicit teaching and learning and at the other extreme some ward rounds containing a substantial amount of training, some of which has been carefully planned and/or followed up.

In this spirit, every ward round should, at its conclusion, offer trainees a chance to put questions to the coach. Even the busiest trainer can afford to offer trainees the 3-minute round-up.

115

> **THE 3-MINUTE ROUND-UP**
>
> If, at the end of the ward round, there is no follow-up phase, the coach says to the trainee(s):
>
> *The next 3 minutes are exclusively yours. You will have my full attention and nothing will interrupt us. Ask me anything at all, either arising from the ward round or your training menu for today or because there is something since we last met that you want to talk about. OK, fire away.*

Trials with this 'round up' indicate that trainees do have questions to ask and points to make, and the 3 minutes will be used up. Of course, the coach may be able to give more than 3 minutes if the questions flow. But where more than 3 minutes cannot be spared, the coach is free to say that time is up, and further questions must be banked until the next round-up.

Here's a trainer explaining the 3-minute round-up to a trainee:

> *Every time we go round on a ward round together, at the end of the round, before we finish, before we go away, we'll stop for 3 minutes — by my watch! That's 3 minutes in which you can ask me anything you like. It's your opportunity to come back on anything that may have happened, either in the ward round or at some other time. It's a little bite of time just for you every time we go round. It will be a guaranteed 3 minutes by the watch, so we're not talking about having long sessions. It's not a lecture or anything. If you haven't got anything to ask me, that's it. I'm not going to volunteer anything at that time. So it's 3 minutes for you to clear up questions or problems that you might have. I'm not talking about service here, that's part of the ward round. Pure training questions. And be ready to remind me about it, don't let me get away with it — no matter what, you get your 3 minutes.*

The value of the 3-minute round-up is that:

- it ensures a teaching element in every ward round, even Type 1
- it reaffirms to trainees that the trainer is taking teaching as a priority
- it gives trainees some 'sacred' space which they value greatly
- it encourages trainees to store up good questions, from the ward round and from elsewhere, and makes sure they are answered before (as is too often their fate) they are forgotten.

## A TRAINEE'S EVALUATION OF THE 3-MINUTE ROUND-UP

*When we did it, it worked out very well. At the end of the ward round or clinic, we'd talk about something we'd just seen or in more general terms as opposed to the specific case that we might have seen. It definitely improved what I got out of the ward rounds and clinics. It gave me more opportunity to ask questions I might not have thought of asking, because you're moving on to the next thing — there's always something waiting for you. If you've got 3 minutes, you have to stop and think 'Oh, I wasn't sure about that point' or 'I understood what we were doing there, but in more general terms what might we have done if this, that and the other?' And all the questions that were there at the back of my mind. We both had things to get on with, but for [the] to stop for 3 minutes, that was definitely helpful.*

## ACTION POINTS ON OJT ON THE WARD

- treat every ward round as, in some ways and at some parts, a teaching round, especially if you have some that are designated teaching rounds

- on each ward round select the type most appropriate to the trainees' needs and the circumstances/pressures prevailing at the time:
  - Type 1 — ward round only (designated teaching or business)
  - Type 2 — planning phase and ward round
  - Type 3 — ward round and follow-up phase
  - Type 4 — planning phase and ward round and follow-up phase

- make sure everybody involved understands why you vary ward round types and don't use the same one every time

- in the planning phase, work out a training menu for the trainee(s) or encourage them to devise one of their own to focus their learning

- use the 3-minute round-up every time

- encourage trainees to remind you about the 3-minute round up in case you forget

- let trainees conduct some ward rounds — but remember that they'll feel discouraged if, without giving reasons, you take over part way through.

# 14 DEVELOPING CLINICAL JUDGEMENT

*Any man who is not positively ham-fisted to begin with can in the end achieve the dexterity to perform safe, sound surgery . . . The decision to operate, when to operate and what operation to do, is in nearly every circumstance more important for the patient's welfare than precisely how the operation is done.*

Sir Hedley Atkins, surgeon, 1977

*The young man knows the rules, but the old man knows the exceptions . . . The young man feels uneasy if he is not continually doing something to stir up a patient's internal arrangements. The old man takes things more quietly and is more willing to let well alone.*

Oliver Wendell Holmes, physician, 1871

## THIS SECTION:

- **examines the concept of clinical judgement**
- **considers problems of how clinical judgement might be acquired or taught**
- **contrasts the concepts of education and training**

From the trainee's point of view, training consists of the progressive acquisition of knowledge, skill and understanding. These three concepts overlap in practice, but they can be distinguished from one another in broad terms. Knowledge is usually easier to acquire than a skill; and a skill is usually easier to acquire than deep understanding. When a given level of knowledge, skill and understanding has been achieved, the trainee is regarded as a competent practitioner.

At the beginning of their postgraduate specialist training, trainees are very conscious of how very much they have still to learn. Over time, as they are given more and more responsibility by Consultants without close supervision, trainees gain in confidence and skill. Few, however, will wish to become merely competent. Many aspire to achieve the highest quality of Consultant practice and to acquire the Consultant's way of thinking, which include:

- wide and extensive experience
- a deep knowledge of a specialty or domain/sub-specialty
- the ability to work more efficiently
- a record of fewer than average errors in diagnostic or management decisions
- a record of better than average outcomes for patients
- the ability to think creatively and critically within the specialist way of thinking

**119**

- sophisticated meta-cognitive skills to think about one's own thinking skills
- a reputation that commands the respect of peers.

Those who, through a combination of talent, experience and favourable opportunities, meet the above criteria, possess a wisdom that goes beyond the acknowledged competence characteristic of the average surgeon. Such wisdom is not so much about technical operating skills but about the making of high quality decisions, including the decision not to operate.

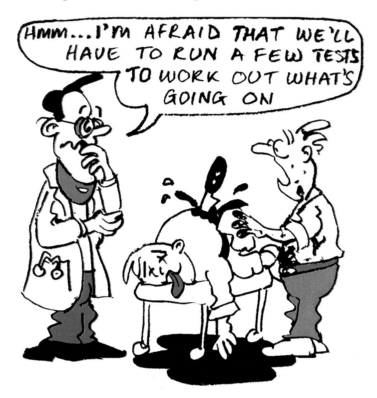

VIEWS OF SOME CONSULTANT SURGEONS (1996)

*The only difference between me and registrars who are good here is that I make better decisions than they do. I know when not to do something. I say, 'Look, you guys: you're young, your brains are better, your eyes are better, your hands are better, so how come I do it better?' The answer's because I make better decisions and I'm more relaxed. The knife, fork and spoon, juniors have to have that, but that's not the heart of it. What they're getting insidiously is an attitude. With experience you learn to sit back and wait and watch and don't treat everything like a protocol or a paradigm. That's the difficult part to teach in medicine. We all want to be at the point where, as it was once said of a great surgeon, 'He made the right decision on the wrong information.'*

*As I mature more in the specialty, I find it easier to turn down some patients who are referred for what is truly inappropriate surgery. I recall a recent case where the patient was very ill and had had a string of previous operations, some of which had failed. People desperately wanted him kept alive. I was under enormous pressure to operate but I feared the patient would probably die under my knife. When I explained this to the family, there was a huge sigh of relief. Nobody had confronted the reality of the situation with them before. They kept being told 'Just one more operation and it'll be all right.' But the truth was he was never going to be all right. He died under the palliative care of a physician with his whole family there in what was a rewarding experience for everybody. If I'd operated, frankly it would have been all blood, guts and glory. I'd probably have emerged from the operating theatre, dripping with sweat saying, 'I'm so very sorry, he didn't make it.' The way I chose, because I'm older and more experienced, was better. Death is a reasonable and acceptable end-point under certain conditions — though this needs considerable consultation and counselling with the relatives and patient concerned.*

**Clinical judgement** is an important aspect of the end-point to which each trainee is striving. It includes:

- the ability to make a competent diagnosis and prognosis and to select an appropriate treatment
- the ability, based on extensive and cumulative experience, to make high quality or expert judgement on a regular basis
- the capacity to reason or make judgements on an intuitive, implicit and 'artistic' basis rather than on an analytical, explicit and 'scientific' basis
- the capacity to deploy, in the interests of a particular patient, evidence-based knowledge to complement personal experience of a condition
- the acquisition of high-level meta-cognitive skills, that is, the ability to monitor, reflect upon and change one's way of thinking and reasoning
- the ability to use research on clinical judgement, reasoning and decision making to enhance one's own capacities in relation to each of these.

*As a trainee, when I came up against a good surgeon there was always more to learn than simply the technical aspects of surgery. There were things not taught in any formal way and I absorbed, almost by osmosis, how he made his judgements. Probably he himself didn't know how he reached it, except that it's an amalgam of academic knowledge and experience in the operating room, in the clinic and on the ward, and the assimilation of the patient's own factors — age, general condition, family background. It's all those things together that finally allow you to make a judgement.*

Consultant surgeon

Clinical judgement is often taken as synonymous with **clinical reasoning** and refers to different cognitive processes.

Sometimes it is used to mean the **hypothetico-deductive** reasoning employed when making a diagnosis, in which the clinician

- collects evidence about the patient's condition — signs and symptoms, etc.
- generates one or more (tentative) hypotheses to account for the observed cues
- interprets the evidence in the light of the hypothesis, which is thereby tested
- evaluates the hypothesis with a view to acceptance, modification or rejection.

Sometimes it is used to mean **pattern recognition**, the **inductive** process by which the clinician recognises, often on an intuitive basis, a pattern in the multiple available data — history, signs and symptoms, X-rays/scans, results of tests and investigations — and thereby reaches a rapid diagnostic conclusion.

Experienced clinicians probably use both approaches to reasoning, but are bound to use hypothesis-testing when no pattern is recognised. Trainees may not know the pattern or be able to apply the pattern recognition strategy, and so fall back on explicit hypothesis-testing far more frequently than does the Consultant.

> We all know surgeons who are technically excellent but whose patients don't do well, because they aren't able to be sure that the operation they're doing is what that patient needs. Some clinicians simply follow an algorithm of disease or treatment. If they have this, I do that, and if they have that, I do the other thing. And it's possible to justify it, perhaps, on pure pathology or anatomy. But the approach is mechanistic. Of course early in their training surgeons have to concentrate on acquiring the necessary skills and techniques. It's only when you've got a grasp of those that you can then start to put it into the context of the patient. In terms of judgement, whether that's the appropriate step in the algorithm to take, that is where the guile comes in. It's very easy to do the right thing for the wrong patient at the wrong time. The best clinicians have this surgical judgement, that something which you just know is the right decision for the patient. Doing the right thing for the right patient for the right reasons at the right time. I once went to a more experienced colleague and asked, 'I have this patient who's suffering from X — who do I send him to?' And the colleague said', Does the patient want an opinion or an operation?'
> Consultant surgeon, 1996

Trainees will meet a number of consultant-coaches who regularly make such wise, high quality decisions. Part of the difficulty is that much OJT is highly fragmented, so that in many surgical specialties relatively few of the most complex cases are followed by junior doctors from initial referral to clinic through to discharge after a stay in hospital. Yet the acquisition of the specialist's way of thinking and of the high level of competence required to make good decisions depends on this holistic view of the patient's medical career.

> The difficult part of surgical training is deciding what to do when, the before and the after, not just the surgery itself. The most important training that's required is in the decision making, not the physical handling. You can teach a monkey how to use the knife. Juniors often think the measure of the quality of their training is the number of cases they've done in theatre. That's not right. They lose sight of the fact that the art of it is the deciding before and after.
>
> Consultant surgeon, 1996

> [In a previous job] I was made to spend almost all my time on the wards and very rarely got into theatre. We saw patients before the surgery and after it, but not the surgery itself.
>
> Trainee, 1996

## Promoting the acquisition of clinical judgement

Clinical judgement is using sophisticated clinical reasoning to reach high quality clinical decisions. Can it be taught? Can it be modelled? Are there other ways in which trainees may be helped to acquire it?

> I don't know whether you can teach judgement — you can show it. And you can learn judgement by watching somebody who has no judgement, so that you can learn judgement without being taught it. I don't think you can teach judgement to a level which one likes to think experts have or consultants have. You can't give a lecture on 'This is clinical judgement, this is clinical guile'. One surgeon I worked for said to me, 'I'm a third rate surgeon: I make up for it with first rate surgical judgement.' I've always remembered that, because it impressed upon me the strength and the power of surgical judgement. The surgeon should be a physician who operates occasionally.
>
> Consultant surgeon, 1996

> Although you have a system and a routine, you've to learn when you have to do it a different way and for a reason. That's hard to teach — when to break your own rules.
>
> Consultant surgeon, 1996

It may be that clinical judgement either cannot be taught in any direct way or can be taught only with great difficulty. However, the trainer can unquestionably create conditions that favour the acquisition of clinical judgement by the trainee.

**123**

The first way of so doing is by **directly structuring** OJT, because it is opportunistic, OJT is naturally fragmented. The coach can compensate for such heavy concentration on the immediate decisions and practical action by deliberately tying these concerns to the patient's wider medical history and career. In other words, the coach ties the immediate events under discussion in an OJT session to the 'before' and the 'after' in a holistic way.

A second way is for the coach to be as explicit as possible about the reasoning behind a judgement or decision or to encourage trainees to talk through what was probably implicit and tacit in the coach's own thinking concerning that judgement or decision. This ties the issue of **evidence and reasoning** (through discussion) to **experience** (through service).

Here are examples of how a coach uses questioning to help trainees acquire clinical judgement. Through the form and content of the question, the coach provides a kind of scaffolding to help trainees to climb to an idea or a mental process that would be impossible for them if left to their own devices.

### QUESTIONS DIRECTED TO PROMOTING CLINICAL JUDGEMENT

*How did you arrive at that diagnosis? Talk me through your reasoning. Did the patient's age and ethnicity influence your thinking?*

*How do you think I made the diagnosis so quickly? What was the pattern I recognised?*

*How do you think I arrived at my diagnosis? Are you convinced it's the right diagnosis? Are there alternatives we should consider? On what grounds should we decide between the two?*

*You are toying with two diagnostic hypotheses. Is there any difference between them in terms of options for management?*

*There are four ways of doing this operation, all of which are widely used. What do you think went through my mind in selecting this particular one for this patient?*

*Of the three consultants in this Department each has a different approach to this operation. Have you worked out yet why we differ on this? Do you think one of these arguments is more persuasive than the others?*

*Would we adopt a different management plan if this were a 20-year-old very active man rather than a rather frail woman of 80?*

*Why do you think this treatment doesn't seem to be working with this patient? Can you think of other patients with whom it might have been more effective? With hindsight, might we have made a better decision?*

A third way is by using the training menu to help the trainee to concentrate and focus learning on just one disease/illness/complaint (or a small number of them) during clinic or a theatre list or ward round. On arrival in the specialty or sub-specialty, the trainee is directed to mastering the relatively simple examples of the most common conditions and their management, which rapidly gives the trainee confidence and of course ensures a more effective early contribution to service. Over time, the coach changes the focus progressively to more complex and rarer conditions and their management.

**Intensive focus** on a limited area allows the coach to help trainees:

- to justify their suggested diagnosis/management (if the suggestion is right, to confirm that the reasoning as well as the conclusion is sound; if the suggestion is wrong, to explore and correct not just the suggestion but the reasoning behind it)
- to explore the process of pattern-recognition, or hypothesis-testing, or both
- to learn that hypothesis-testing is a way forward if a pattern cannot be recognised
- to think out several hypotheses rather than being stuck with the first one they think of
- to test the most obvious hypothesis first, and to look for disconfirming as well as supportive evidence
- to check all the hypotheses as fully and systematically as possible to prevent premature closure on a favoured hypothesis
- to learn that ruling out one hypothesis may rule out others too — hypotheses can be nested and tested in logical and economical ways
- to examine a range of management options and their appropriateness to the characteristics and circumstances of the patient.

## Education and training: creating a training culture

Novices expect to be trained: they want the knowledge, techniques and skills that mark the competent medical practitioner, and training, both on and off the job, is an appropriate way of obtaining them. Novices' attitudes to their learning and the way they are taught tend to be short-term, specific, instrumental, utilitarian, extrinsic — the demands of the next examination, the next post, the next operation, the next day.

In the later stages of the Specialist Registrar grade, with examinations happily past and most of the core knowledge, techniques and skills of the specialty or sub-specialty in one's grasp, the trainee's outlook inclines more favourably to education rather than training — learning that emphasises the longer-term, the complex, understanding rather than knowledge, the problem or the solution that is intrinsically interesting rather than immediately useful. At the same time, there is, to the eye of the experienced Consultant, the danger of over-confidence.

> In a Registrar there can be a level of confidence that in retrospect I recognise in myself, which wasn't appropriate or justified, despite the training. Everybody goes through it, undoubtedly: you think you've got the basic skills, you've mastered highly specialised skills. That's when you're most dangerous and are at risk of doing something stupid.
>
> Experienced Consultant

Newly appointed Consultants usually acknowledge that they have much to learn.

> There are some procedures I've done less of and still need to consolidate as a Consultant, even though one of the juniors working with me may be quite capable of doing it. It's my role to make sure that no juniors assisting me or working under my supervision get into any difficulty that I can't get them out of. So I have to become a master of the whole operation before I can give key parts of it away to my assistant as part of his training.
>
> Newly appointed Consultant

It is for this reason that the early years of the Consultant's first post are so important in the development of clinical judgement, reasoning and decision making.

> Judgement is a very difficult thing to teach. It's one thing that young Consultants can have a problem with because of our consultancy system. I would say the ones who come here take 3 years to be a Consultant. We have this business in Britain of all Consultants being equal, which is patently rubbish. It encourages surgeons go through the pupa stage of Senior Registrar and then expect suddenly to be transformed into the wondrous butterfly of a Consultant. Some then find it difficult to talk to their colleagues, to ask advice and say: 'How do I do this?' or continue to train in judgement. Some take time to adjust. Others happily don't, and are very good at it.
>
> Experienced Consultant surgeon

# The effects of a training culture

A group of Consultants who see themselves as learners and who are committed to the training of their juniors create a culture of training, in which it is evident that learning is highly valued and a natural concomitant to high quality service. When service is seen by the coaches as a source of learning for themselves, it will be so seen by trainees, and the simplistic antithesis between 'training' (i.e. uninterrupted by service) and 'service' (i.e. which excludes training) is defeated. Training can be dry and difficult to apply when it is divorced from practice; service can simply be 'work' when it is disconnected from learning. A learning culture does not necessarily mean more formal teaching or more direct supervision by consultants or a lower service commitment from trainees. It means that the environment is one in which **opportunities for learning** and the **importance of learning** pervade the work of all, whether the activity be called service, on-the-job training or formal training. It also means that coaches and trainees seek a balance between critical discussion *What are we doing for what reasons?* and the experience of continual service.

The acquisition of clinical judgement by the Specialist Registrar is an important objective in the education of a surgeon. It is in this area of improving judgement through OJT that the closest professional bond is created between Consultant and trainee. The most outstanding coaches, through their infectious enthusiasm for their work, their commitment to teaching and their willingness to share their expertise, undoubtedly educate as well as train their juniors. They openly continue to learn — from any source. It is with good reason that the later stages of learning in medicine are usually referred to as continuing medical education (CME), which is aided by growing experience and the on-the-job learning that is enhanced by training others.

It is this change in the culture that plays such an important role in transforming training into education. Effective OJT, in which service is the medium of training, is the principal structural support of an educational environment and training culture in which everybody learns.

**127**

# 15 CONCLUSION

The environment in which surgeons are trained is changing. Hospitals are busier and increasingly driven by the need to meet service contracts; the period of training is shorter; and hours of work are restricted.

These changes should be seen as an opportunity to improve postgraduate surgical training, not an obstacle to it. In order to do so, surgeons should consider striking a new balance between the various approaches to teaching and learning:

- formal and didactic teaching, presentations, seminars etc.
- journal clubs
- courses
- personal and private study
- on-the-job training
- research and audit.

Effective OJT is assuming greater importance. Changing from apprenticeship-by-osmosis to apprenticeship-by-coaching poses the greatest challenge. Effective OJT requires a distinctive relationship between coach and trainee, and this has five principal features.

- the coach makes maximal use of the opportunities for teaching that become available during service
- the trainee is pro-active in a similar search for, and use of, learning opportunities and is skilful in eliciting teaching from the coach
- the coach is skilled in selecting an appropriate teaching technique (questioning, explaining, demonstrating etc.) in a particular setting (theatre, ward, clinic) for a chosen training focus (the training menu of the day) within a progressive sequence of training (the training plan)
- there is regular feedback provided in a variety of forms. The trainee has a strong sense of progression in learning and a record of it
- training is minimally disruptive of service delivery because wherever possible OJT is fusional.

The various forms of OJT are at the centre of surgical training because they link training to patient care. The close relationship between OJT and service delivery offers the opportunity for the development of, and education in, the most elusive of surgical skills — judgement. The challenge to both consultants and specialist registrars is to make the changes necessary for creating the high quality OJT that can play such a key role in the training of surgeons.

> *New ideas build their nests in young men's brains.*
>
> Oliver Wendell Holmes, physician, 1871

# ACKNOWLEDGEMENTS

The University of Cambridge Training of Doctors in Hospitals Project is sponsored by the Postgraduate Dean, Dr JSG Biggs, and funded by the Anglia Postgraduate Medical and Dental Education Committee.

We acknowledge with gratitude the assistance and advice of the following, who contributed to the ideas, the development of practice, the field-testing and criticism of the emerging text. We are of course entirely responsible for the shortcomings of the work.

## Consultant Surgeons

David Conlan, Christopher Constant, David Dandy, John Dunning, Dennis Edwards, Charles Galasko, Stephen Large, Clare Marx, Samer Nashef, Murray Matthewson, Hugh Phillips, Andrew Ritchie, John Wallwork, Francis Wells

## Specialist Registrars/Senior Registrars

Ahmed Arifi, Clifford Barlow, Peter Bobak, Peter Braidley, John Calder, Simon Carney, Jonathan Hobby, James Hopkinson-Wooley, Reza Hosseinpour, Tim Mitchell, Fabian Norman-Taylor, Fred Robinson, Stephen Tsui, Simon Ward, Tern Wilmink

## Senior House Officers

Cheryl Baldwick, Jason Braybrooke, Damian Fahy, Matthew Gaskarth, Michael Green, Charles Imber, Juliet King, Harry Parissis, David Redfern, Gabriel Sayer, Michael Schenker, Gunther Selzer

## Project Team Members

Joy Anderson, Martin Booth, Howard Bradley, Geoff Southworth, Paula Stanley

# BIOGRAPHY

David H Hargreaves is Professor of Education at the University of Cambridge and a Fellow of Wolfson College. He is a Director of the University of Cambridge Project on the Training of Doctors in Hospitals and the author of numerous books and articles in learned journals on professional and institutional development.

Mark G Bowditch is Specialist Registrar in Orthopaedic and Trauma Surgery on the Cambridge and East Anglian Training Programme. He studied Physiology and Medicine at the University of Manchester. He has been a lecturer in Anatomy in Glasgow and is involved in undergraduate and postgraduate training in Cambridge. He is associated with the University of Cambridge Project on the Training of Doctors in Hospitals.

Damian R Griffin is a Specialist Registrar in Orthopaedic and Trauma Surgery on the Cambridge and East Anglian Training Programme and an associate Fellow of Gonville and Caius College. He studied Physiology at Cambridge and Clinical Medicine in Oxford. He has been involved in teaching undergraduates and in postgraduate training at the Royal College of Surgeons in London. He is associated with the University of Cambridge Project on the Training of Doctors in Hospitals.